THE THYROID
SOURCEBOOK

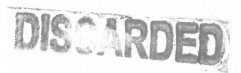

Other books by M. Sara Rosenthal

The Gynecological Sourcebook (1994, Lowell House)
The Pregnancy Sourcebook (1994, Lowell House)
The Fertility Sourcebook (1995, Lowell House)
The Breastfeeding Sourcebook (1995, Lowell House)
The Breast Sourcebook (1996, Lowell House)

The Thyroid Sourcebook

Everything You Need to Know

Second Edition

M. Sara Rosenthal

with a foreword by
Robert Volpé, M.D., F.R.C.P., F.A.C.P.

Lowell House
Los Angeles

Contemporary Books
Chicago

To my maternal grandparents
Jacob Lander, M.D. (1910–1989)
Clara Lander, Ph.D. (1916–1978)

Library of Congress Cataloging-in-Publication Data

Rosenthal, M. Sara
  The thyroid sourcebook : everything you need to know / M. Sara Rosenthal.
    p.   cm.
  Includes bibliographical references and index.
  ISBN 1-56565-482-X
  1. Thyroid gland—Popular works. I. Title.
RC655.R67 1993
616.4'4—dc20   93-10425
                                                          CIP

Requests for such permissions should be addressed to:
Lowell House
2029 Century Park East, Suite 3290
Los Angeles, CA 90067

Publisher: Jack Artenstein
Associate Publisher, Lowell House Adult: Bud Sperry
Text design: Mary Ballachino/Merrimac Design

Manufactured in the United States of America
10 9 8 7 6 5 4 3 2

Acknowledgments

If it weren't for the commitment, hard work and guidance of the following people, this book would never have been written: Robert Volpé, M.D., F.R.C.P. (C), who served as Medical Adviser; Rosemary Powers, R.N., M.Sc.N., who served as research assistant; my Editor, Janice Gallagher; and my copyeditor, Dianne J. Woo.

Special thanks to the physicians and health practitioners who donated their time and expertise: Gillian Arsenault, M.Sc., M.D., I.B.C.L.C.; Pamela H. Craig, M.D., F.A.C.S.; Daniel Drucker, M.D., F.R.C.P. (C); Heather Dawson, M.D., C.C.F.P.; Susan R. George, M.D., F.R.C.P. (C), F.A.C.P.; Leslie M.C. Goldenberg, M.D., F.R.C.P. (C); Masood A. Khatamee, M.D., F.A.C.O.G.; Matthew Lazar, M.D., F.R.C.P. (C), F.A.C.P; Suzanne Pratt, M.D., F.A.C.O.G.; Bob Pritchard, B.Sc.PMH.; Daniel Rappaport, M.D., F.R.C.P.(C); and Irving B. Rosen, M.D., F.R.C.S. (C), F.A.C.S.; Douglas Ross, Senior Product Manager, Knoll Pharma Inc.; Sharon Wyman-Cunningham, Product Manager, Franklin Diagnostics, Inc.

Finally, in the moral support department—my husband, Gary S. Karp, and all the relatives and friends who cheered me on.

Contents

Foreword

The Thyroid Sourcebook is intended primarily for persons with thyroid disease. The book came out of the author's own experience in which she had to deal with a thyroid condition and felt she required more information. In her discussions with other patients she found that many were concerned that they had not obtained a full understanding of their condition; some were unsatisfied about the time taken to make the diagnosis, about the care they received, and about continued problems that they attributed to their thyroid abnormality. Some of these perceptions are not fully representative of the majority of patients' experiences; nevertheless, they are valid and must be dealt with in a sensitive and compassionate fashion. Moreover, it is important for patients to have a full comprehension of their disorders at their individual level of understanding. It is possible that some physicians do not take the time or do not express themselves in appropriate language to make the patient's entry into the thyroid world an easy one. Ms. Rosenthal's descriptions of the various thyroid conditions are certainly nontechnical, and they convey an image of thyroid disease that might not be found in a book written by an endocrinologist or a general physician. The book thus reflects the feelings experienced by patients with thyroid conditions and may give them insight into the types of questions that would be appropriate to ask their physician. In this sense, the book is a good introduction for patients with thyroid disease, and helps inquisitive patients learn more about the maladies that are affecting them.

Robert Volpé, M.D., F.R.C.P., F.A.C.P
Professor, Department of Medicine
University of Toronto

Introduction:
The Book I Had to Write

The inspiration to write *The Thyroid Sourcebook* came from the women in my family: from my great-grandmother who developed a goiter in the 1930s; from my grandmother, who developed Graves' disease in 1940 with her first pregnancy at age 24, had her thyroid removed, and subsequently was not given any medication because her doctor said she "didn't need it"; from my mother, who developed Graves' disease in 1981, watched in dismay as her eyes bulged out like *her* mother's did, and read through stacks of complicated medical texts to try to find out more about her illness; from my aunt, who became severely hypothyroid in her late thirties, and her daughter, who developed thyroid cancer at age 20; and from my older sister, who in 1991 had to beg her family doctor for a thyroid test on her thirtieth birthday because she knew thyroid disorders "run in the family." Her doctor reluctantly ordered the test and was surprised to find out she, too, had Graves' disease.

Statistically, my family's thyroid heritage is not remarkable. In 1983, when I turned 20, my family's "legacy" was passed down to me as well: I was diagnosed with thyroid cancer. Within a short span of months, my thyroid gland and the lymph nodes on the right side of my neck were surgically removed. I was then required to drink radioactive iodine from a lead container a couple of times. During my final treatment stage, I visited a hospital basement for external radiation therapy every morning for an entire month. On my 21st birthday I was given the "all clear." But I was never given any information about what I had gone through and would continue to live with.

I had to rely on relatives and friends of friends who were doctors for basic "what's a thyroid?" information. I flirted with the interns so that I could be privy to juicy facts and tidbits on the thyroid gland, and I was reduced to eavesdropping on my surgeon (while he was examining me) as he outlined my history and prognosis to the troupe of medical students accompanying him on his rounds. One day I rudely interrupted his lecture and dared to ask him a question. Everyone looked surprised, and one student asked me if I was "in sciences." Patients should be seen and not heard was the message.

After my thyroidectomy I went to my surgeon to get my stitches removed. At that point I asked him if he could spare a few moments to answer some questions. His eyes widened as I produced a list of about 40 questions, carefully written out the night before. This time he got *my* message.

The point is, nobody should have to go through what my family and I did without guidance and information. That's why I wrote this book. This is *your* thyroid book.

The truth is, for every 20 people in the world, at least one has developed or will develop a thyroid disorder. In fact, over 13 million people in the United States and Canada alone suffer from thyroid disorders—and 9 million of them are women. Thyroid disorders occur five to seven times more frequently in women. Because of this, not only have I written in detail about the thyroid gland, the disorders and diseases that affect it (chapters 1–6), and the symptoms and treatments of each disorder (chapters 1–6 and 11), but I've also included a thorough discussion of how thyroid disorders uniquely affect women and men.

In chapter 7, I've provided the most current information on thyroid dysfunction during pregnancy and menopause, as well as information on the use of various contraceptive pills while on thyroid replacement hormone. Chapter 7 also discusses a phenomenon known as Hiroshima Maiden syndrome, a term that refers to women who have developed thyroid disorders as a direct result of electrolysis. Meanwhile, I also discuss the issue of women misusing thyroid medication for the purposes of weight control.

Chapter 8 is for the men out there coping with thyroid disorders. I've included the latest facts on how thyroid disorders affect the male physique and men emotionally.

Chapter 9 discusses how thyroid disorders can affect children.

Retardation and cretinism are classic consequences of an undiagnosed thyroid problem in infants and children.

Finally, I've included information on the emotional issues associated with the symptoms, diagnosis, and treatment of thyroid disease and other disorders. In particular, new information on depression related to hypothyroidism is outlined in chapter 2, and chapter 10, entitled "A Layperson's Guide to Doctors," provides guidance in choosing and dealing with doctors at all levels of specialization. Chapter 12 is devoted to thyroid medication and balancing other medications with it. It also provides guidance in choosing and dealing with pharmacists. Chapter 13 is a wrap-up discussion covering issues such as nutrition, thyroid "maintenance," and research.

To write this book I interviewed thyroid specialists, endocrinologists, nuclear medicine practitioners, radiotherapists, pharmacists, head and neck surgeons, family practitioners, gynecologists and obstetricians, oncologists, gerontologists, pediatricians, social workers and psychiatrists, radiologists, and dozens of thyroid patients across the United States and Canada. I also researched complex medical texts and documents not published for consumer use.

If you suffer from thyroid disease or any related disorders, remember that you're not alone. This book is intended to give you important information explained in nontechnical language as well as guidance and support. Read it, use it, and share it with other thyroid sufferers.

Introduction to the Second Edition: You've Truly Made this *Your* Thyroid Sourcebook

Welcome to the second edition of *The Thyroid Sourcebook*. As I mentioned in the previous introduction, the inspiration to write this came from my own battle with misinformation and the lack of information about what I was going through as a thyroid patient. But, I stressed that this book was written for *you;* it was always meant to be *your* thyroid sourcebook.

When the first edition was published, it was exactly 10 years after my thyroid surgery and treatment. I wasn't sure how people were going to respond to medical information provided in such plain, nontechnical language. Though, I was also convinced that there was a need for a thorough book written by a thyroid patient for a thyroid patient. As a journalist and someone who has experienced every imaginable test and treatment, I took up the task, and then, my readers continued to pass this torch on. Today, I get calls and letters from those who have benefited from my book in ways I never dreamed possible. In fact, the revisions and updates in this edition are inspired by readers' experiences, not my own. I've kept notes from telephone conversations, letters, and e-mail, and you hold in your hands thyroid experiences from across the continent (and many from Great Britain).

So what's new? You'll find the latest information on smoking and thyroid eye disease; osteoporosis and thyroid hormone; post-partum thyroid disease; nutrition and diet (an area that women on thyroid hormone replacement especially requested); the continuing problem of iodine deficiency around the world; as well as an expanded section on hyper- and hypothyroid symptoms discussed alphabetically under the "Hyperalphabet Soup" and the "Hypoalphabet Soup" sections in chapter 2. Of particular interest may be the new sections in the "doctor chapter" (chapter 10), where I discuss the many areas of mismanagement of this disease. I also refer you to "The Long Half-Life of Radioactive Myths" in chapter 11; an expanded chapter on thyroid medication in chapter 12; as well as an expanded section on thyroid research and the future of thyroid disease. In short, with few exceptions, every chapter of this book has been completely revised and updated. I've exhausted the medical literature for which tests and treatments are appropriate in the late 1990s, and which are obsolete. I've even provided some illustrations this time around, which I hope you'll find useful.

Finally the resource list has been vastly expanded to include Internet instructions, websites, thyroid organizations from around the world (many of which were formed after the publication of the first edition), including information on the Thyroid Federation International, a newly-formed consortium of international thyroid organizations, of which I am a founding member.

As you read this book, I will be busy looking into new issues for the next edition, issues such as thyroid disease incidence and AIDS—an area that was difficult to find enough information for this edition. Remember, this is still your thyroid sourcebook. It always will be.

Meet Your Thyroid Gland

Whether you've just been diagnosed with a thyroid disorder, treated for one long ago, or suspect a thyroid problem, it's important first to understand what the thyroid gland actually *does* in the body. Generally, when we hear the word *thyroid,* all kinds of words flash before our eyes: *fat, goiter, bulgy eyes, metabolism, iodine.* It is how these fragments fit into the larger picture that is confusing.

The purpose of this chapter is to make the pieces fit. It describes where the thyroid gland is located, what it does, and how it works. It also explains how the thyroid gland can malfunction and why, addresses some of the myths we've heard about the thyroid gland, and differentiates between the myths and facts. Finally, this chapter outlines some of the ways you can trace thyroid disorders in your family.

Since this chapter serves as a general introduction to the thyroid gland, it will continuously refer you ahead to other chapters in the book for more details. The idea is to provide you with enough information about the thyroid gland so you can fully participate in making diagnosis and treatment decisions.

How Your Thyroid Works

Think of your body as a small country. It lives off its own natural resources and domestic produce, it exports its surplus goods, and it imports fundamental materials for its own use.

An import would be anything not naturally present in your body, such as food and oxygen. An export is anything the body naturally manufactures in surplus, such as protein, fat, and secretions. For example, sweat, urine, and skin are daily exports; every day you dispose of bodily wastes by shedding dead skin cells, blowing your nose, sweating, and urinating. Finally, a domestic product is anything your body naturally manufactures and *keeps*, such as hormones and white blood cells.

Your thyroid gland is a crucial domestic manufacturer. It is located in the lower part of your neck, in front of your windpipe, and the products it makes are two thyroid hormones—thyroxine, known as T_4 (four iodine atoms), and triiodothyronine, known as T_3 (three

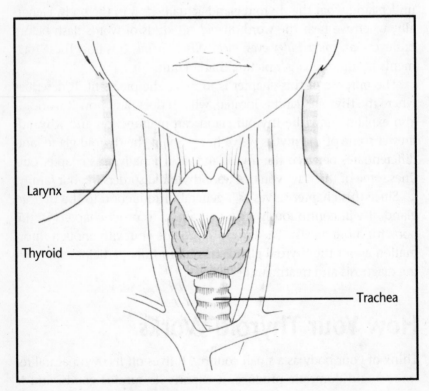

Fig. 1-1 Where your thyroid lives.

Reprinted from *Nichts Gutes im Schilde Krankheiten der Schilddruse.* Copyright 1994, Georg Thieme Publishing.

iodine atoms). Thyroid hormone (the two hormones are referred to in the singular) is then secreted into the circulation and becomes widely distributed throughout the body; it is one of the basic regulators of the functions of every cell and every tissue within the body, and a steady supply is crucial for good health.

The thyroid gland is not totally self-sufficient, however; it needs to import one key ingredient for production: iodine. Your thyroid gland extracts iodine from various foods, including certain vegetables, shellfish, milk products (cow udders are washed with large amounts of iodine, which ends up in your milk), and anything with iodized salt. Normally, we take in sufficient iodine through our diet.

Our thyroids are very sensitive to iodine. When the thyroid gland is not able to obtain sufficient quantities of iodine, you can develop what is called a goiter, or enlarged thyroid. A goiter can also develop if your thyroid gland absorbs too much iodine and produces either too little or too much thyroid hormone. Although it seems odd that too much or too little iodine can produce the same results, the reason the goiter develops in each case is different. Too little iodine can cause increased activity of thyroid gland cells, and too much iodine can cause the thyroid gland to enlarge.

Goiter Belts and Iodine Deficiency

A goiter belt is not a fashion accessory. You may be familiar with the term *goiter belt,* which refers to regions in which inhabitants typically suffer from insufficient iodine. The Great Lakes region, for example, was once considered a goiter belt. But the problem of iodine deficiency is far from solved in other parts of the world. In fact, over one billion people are at risk for iodine deficiency-related thyroid disease. Two-hundred million people suffer from goiters, while 20 million people suffer from brain damage due to iodine deficiency in pregnancy and infancy. This is very disturbing, since these problems can be completely prevented by the simple addition of iodized salt or iodized oil (proposed in some regions) to the diet.

The first International Goiter Congress was held in 1929 in Bern after Switzerland and the U.S. introduced iodized salt. Many countries soon followed suit and iodine deficiency has disappeared in most parts of the world. However, not much happened to eliminate iodine deficiency in underdeveloped nations until 1985, when thyroid specialists established the International Council for Control of Iodine Deficiency Disorders (ICCIDD), a group of about 400 members from 70 different countries.

While in North America, only about 1 in 4,000 newborns is born with hypothyroidism, in iodine-deficient areas, 10% of all newborns are hypothyroid. Worse, up to 70% of the iodine-deficient populations are severely hypothyroid. As a result, iodine deficiency is now recognized as the most common cause of preventable mental defects. ICCIDD works with the World Health Organization and UNICEF to develop national programs in Africa, Asia, Latin America, and Europe with the goal of eliminating iodine deficiency by the year 2,000. Most recently, the salt industry has joined in the fight, too.

The Role of Calcitonin

Your thyroid gland rents space to non-thyroid cells called C cells, which make the hormone calcitonin. This hormone helps to regulate calcium and, hence, helps to prevent osteoporosis. But to your *bones*, calcitonin is kind of like a "tonsil." It serves a useful purpose, but when the hormone is not manufactured due to the absence of a thyroid gland (if it's removed or ablated by radioactive iodine), you won't really notice any effects, just as you don't "miss" your tonsils. Calcium levels are really controlled by the parathyroid glands, discussed further on, and is much more dependent on the hormone estrogen, which helps with calcium absorption, diet, and exercise, which builds bone mass.

Calcitonin is only important when discussing the thyroid if you're screening for a rare type of thyroid cancer called medullary thyroid cancer (see chapter 6). When this kind of thyroid cancer develops, your thyroid overproduces calcitonin, which is the telltale marker for this type of cancer. Once the thyroid is removed due to medullary thyroid cancer, continued calcitonin secretions are a sign that not enough thyroid tissue was removed.

The Role of Thyroglobulin

Although this sounds like a Halloween candy, thyroglobulin is a specific protein made only by your thyroid cells, used mostly by the thyroid gland itself to make thyroid hormone. Like calcitonin, this substance isn't all that important to your body once your thyroid is gone; you won't miss it. The only role thyroglobulin plays after your thyroid problem is treated is in screening for thyroid cancer *recurrence*. You see, when your thyroid gland is removed due to any type of thyroid cancer (see chapter 6), this protein should not be manufactured anymore. If thyroglobulin shows up on a blood test, it's a sign that some thyroid tissue was left that is now "active" and, hence, potentially cancerous. For hyperthyroid or hypothyroid patients, however, screening for thyroglobulin is useless.

Things that Can Go Wrong

Like other manufacturers, your thyroid gland is particularly sensitive to the law of supply and demand. Because it isn't licensed to *export* anything at all, it is forced to use everything it produces, suffering the consequences of either overproduction or underproduction.

If, for example, your thyroid gland manufactures too much thyroid hormone, your body will speed up. Your heart rate will increase, and you might feel hot all the time, have diarrhea, lose weight, feel dizzy or shaky. In a sense, the thyroid *eats the costs* at your body's expense. This is known as hyperthyroidism (*hyper* means "too much") and is explained more thoroughly in chapter 2.

If your thyroid manufactures too little hormone, your body suffers immediate losses. Most bodily functions slow right down. You'll have an unusually slow pulse, you'll feel very tired, and you'll have no energy. You might be constipated, you might get a little puffy, you might feel cold all the time, and your skin might get very dry. This is known as hypothyroidism (*hypo* means "too little"), which is also explained in detail in chapter 2.

Your thyroid is under a lot of pressure to meet exact demand for a product it monopolizes. That's where your pituitary gland comes in. It controls and regulates all bodily functions and secretions. The pituitary gland (often referred to as the master gland) is situated at the base of the skull and is, without question, the most influential gland in your body. Your thyroid gland reports directly to it.

The pituitary gland regularly monitors T_4 and T_3 stock in your body's blood levels. When stock is low, it sends a message to your thyroid gland in the form of a stimulating hormone called TSH (thyroid stimulating hormone) and orders it to produce more. The pituitary gland will only secrete increased amounts of TSH when T_4 and/or T_3 levels are low. When hormone levels are adequate, TSH production is quite small; when hormone levels are too high, the pituitary gland stops all TSH secretion. This should alert the thyroid to stop production, but it doesn't always work, particularly when the thyroid gland is infiltrated or under attack.

This situation occurs, for instance, with a multinodular goiter, which is a bumpy or lumpy enlarged thyroid gland. What happens here is that for some unknown reason, a lump or nodule forms on your thyroid gland, mimicking the gland in every conceivable way. These nodules are "wanna-be" thyroid glands. They watch the thyroid gland in action, and in time learn to manufacture T_3 and T_4 as well. They are completely unaware of the pituitary gland, which of course has no knowledge that these nodules exist. The pituitary gland stops secreting TSH, which alerts the thyroid gland to slow down production. But T_3 and T_4 are still being produced in uncontrolled quantities by the copycat nodes. The system breaks down, and you end up hyperthyroid.

This same scenario can take place if you suffer from Graves' disease, which is an autoimmune or self-attacking disease, explained more thoroughly in chapter 3. Here, your body turns on itself. With Graves' disease, the body attacks its very own thyroid gland. Something goes haywire in the immune system, and the thyroid gland is suddenly seen as an enemy. An armed antibody, called thyroid stimulating antibody (TSA) is produced. TSA is then sent on a special search and destroy mission and launches a surprise attack on your poor thyroid gland, which is only doing its job. The result is a communication breakdown between the thyroid gland and the pituitary gland. Confused and disoriented, the thyroid gland makes thyroid hormone like it's going out of style. The pituitary gland again stops TSH secretion, thinking its command to slow down will be obeyed by the thyroid gland. But the thyroid gland's factory has been bombed by attacking TSA forces, and it doesn't read. Once again, you end up hyperthyroid.

So, like any checks-and-balances system, there's always a hole. When your thyroid is out of control, there's no way your body can manage the situation without outside intervention. If it could, all it would have to do is excrete all excess thyroid hormone. Unfortunately, it's not that easy. As a result, overproduction or underproduction of thyroid hormone can cause both structural and functional damage.

Graves' disease is a good example of a thyroid disorder from a *functional* perspective. In the early stages of Graves' disease, the thyroid might enlarge only slightly and perhaps would not be detected by your doctor. To the doctor, your thyroid appears normal in size and shape but scores low in the performance category, overproducing thyroid hormone and causing your body to overwork itself. Performance in this case is measured by a blood test.

A goiter is an example of a *structural* disorder. (Goiters can be caused by Graves' disease or other conditions causing underproduction or overproduction of thyroid hormone.) In this case, your thyroid would actually grow noticeably larger in appearance, something your doctor could definitely verify by simply feeling your neck. For example, if the goiter is a by-product of an overactive thyroid, a blood test may determine hyperthyroidism *before* the goiter grows too large. But many times an overactive thyroid gland isn't diagnosed by your doctor until the enlargement is so pronounced that the doctor can't miss it.

Your thyroid gland is also vulnerable to a hostile takeover. For usually unknown reasons (in some cases exposure to radiation is a cause, which is discussed in chapter 5), the tissue and cells in the thyroid gland mutate and start to reproduce in the form of lumps. These lumps or "cold" nodules are primitive cells that lack the intelligence to produce thyroid hormone. They mindlessly reproduce and mutate without any purpose or direction. (Nodules are discussed in detail in chapter 5.)

When these cold nodules develop, it is not your thyroid gland that is in immediate danger, but the rest of your body. When these nodules appear, their rate of reproduction can increase and spread throughout your body. This is known as thyroid cancer, which is explained in great detail in chapter 6. Ironically, a person with thyroid cancer normally has perfect thyroid function. Usually, when thyroid cancer is detected, surgical removal of your thyroid gland is performed to prevent the spread of the primitive cells. However, many thyroid cancers are very slow-growing and may not spread elsewhere for several years.

The scenarios described above are among the more common thyroid disorders diagnosed. What's important to remember is that thyroid disease is extremely treatable. Even a disorder in the most severe stage can be easily treated or reversed. (However, in this day and age of advanced medicine, it's highly unlikely that any thyroid disorder would reach a severe stage.) The more you understand about the delicate balance necessary for normal thyroid function, the easier it is to grasp how little it takes to upset this balance.

A Word About the Parathyroid Glands

Everyone has at least four parathyroid glands that control the blood calcium level, or calcium balance. (Some people have more than four!) These glands are located on the back of each lobe of your thyroid gland. The easiest way to grasp exactly where they're located is to imagine the capital letter H. At each tip of the H, imagine a circle. If the H is your thyroid gland, the circles at each tip are your parathyroid glands.

Parathyroid glands usually come into play only when you undergo *surgical* treatment for a thyroid condition. Surgery is most commonly required when thyroid cancer is diagnosed or when a goiter resulting from hyperthyroidism has grown out of control.

Because the glands are so close in proximity to the thyroid gland, surgical complications could be serious. Essentially, a surgeon who is performing a thyroidectomy (removal of the thyroid gland), or simply removing benign or malignant growths on or around the thyroid gland, must be careful not to touch or disrupt the parathyroid glands. As long as there is one good functioning parathyroid gland, there's no problem. However, these small glands are susceptible to either temporary or permanent damage during thyroid surgery.

If the parathyroid glands were accidentally removed or damaged from thyroid surgery, your blood calcium levels would drop. This could cause muscle spasms and contractions, seizures or convulsions, and cataracts. If the damage was temporary, you'd need to take calcium intravenously and orally. In the case of permanent damage, you may need to take calcium supplements as well as vitamin D, which helps your body absorb calcium, for the rest of your life, and have your calcium levels checked and tested frequently.

Sometimes, however, tumors can develop on the parathyroid gland itself. These tumors are usually located behind the thyroid gland and do not affect it. When this happens, surgical removal of the parathyroid gland tumor is done. Depending on whether the growths are benign (noncancerous) or malignant (cancerous, which is *rare*), removal of one or more of the parathyroid glands is sometimes necessary. Tumors of the parathyroid are rare and statistically occur in patients who received some form of radiation to their neck in childhood. (See chapter 5 for more detail.)

Thyroid Folklore

Because thyroid hormone affects your entire metabolism, you've probably heard all kinds of rumors and myths about the thyroid gland from a variety of sources. It's important to separate fact from fiction. Hypothyroidism in particular seems to be the cause for the majority of these half-truths.

The most common myth in this weight-obsessed era is the belief that a thyroid problem makes you fat. *This is not true.* The myth arose from the general assumption that if your thyroid is under-active, you gain weight more easily. The fact is, all body types, shapes, and weights can experience hypothyroidism; some hypothyroid people are thin, some are fat. Obesity is caused by eating more food than your body requires, and the reason this occurs usually has more to do with dietary habits and psychological roots. The simple fact is that when you're hypothyroid, your body's metabolism slows down. Unless you change your eating habits to adjust to your slower metabolism, you'll gain weight. The problem that we all encounter is that it's difficult to adjust our intake because in North America we eat for pleasure instead of nourishment. As a result, we suffer the consequences of weight gain.

When you're hypothyroid, the idea is to eat until you don't feel hungry anymore, instead of overstuffing yourself with quantities of food a person with normal thyroid function could handle. In fact, when you're diagnosed with hypothyroidism, the worst thing you can do is suddenly go on a panic diet and deprive yourself of food. This will only make things worse. When your body is deprived of food, it actually becomes more efficient and requires less food to function. This is how the body protects itself from famine and star-vation. Deprivation diets work against you because after you're treated and resume normal thyroid function, you could actually gain weight consuming the same quantity of food before you were hypothyroid. Some nutritionists refer to weight gain caused by de-privation diets as the "yo-yo syndrome." Managing your weight when you're hypothyroid has more to do with being conscious of food than with controlling your intake of it.

Although obesity is statistically considered a common condition in North America, hypothyroidism is not. Fewer than one in 100 obese people are hypothyroid.

Overweight children are also commonly tested for hypothy-roidism but are rarely found to have it. There is a clear difference between a child who is overfed and one who is hypothyroid. For the record, an overfed child is usually tall, while a hypothyroid child is short and will often have a goiter.

Another myth high on the folklore list is the belief that if you're tired or fatigued, you must have a thyroid problem. This also is not true. Although fatigue is often one of many hypothyroid symptoms, it is not by itself a sure sign of hypothyroidism. Fatigue is attributed to an almost infinite variety of causes, including stress, viruses, age, and certain activities.

Here are a few more popular myths that can be put to rest:

MYTH: *Taking thyroid hormone increases fertility.*
FACT: This is only true if your infertility is the direct result of a hyper- or hypothyroid condition. For the record, the chief cause of female infertility is a structural problem, such as blocked fallopian tubes; while the chief cause of male infertility is also structural, often due to blockages within the male reproductive tract. When infertility is caused by a male or female hormonal disorder, only a small fraction of these disorders are due to a thyroid problem. Nevertheless, since thyroid function tests are noninvasive and easy to read, get your doctor to order one if you're having trouble conceiving. For more information about infertility, consult my book *The Fertility Sourcebook*, and see also chapter 7.

MYTH: *Irregular periods mean you have a thyroid condition.*
FACT: Menstruation can certainly be affected by hypothyroidism or hyperthyroidism, but unless changes in your flow or cycle are accompanied by other symptoms (of either hypo- or hyperthyroidism), it's not likely that menstrual disruptions point to a definite thyroid problem. If you are hypothyroid, periods tend to be prolonged and heavy; if you are hyperthyroid, you usually will have scanty periods. Once these thyroid conditions are corrected, however, cycles and flows return to normal. Yet women with perfectly normal thyroid

function can suffer from a host of menstrual ailments that include irregular cycles, irregular flows, and severe cramps. The causes of menstrual abnormalities vary tremendously and can be related to stress, infections, early pregnancy (i.e., a clue that you're pregnant), or signs of menopause. See a gynecologist if you notice abnormal menstrual cycles. Chapter 7 provides more details on this subject.

MYTH: *All short people have thyroid conditions.*

FACT: Undiagnosed hypothyroidism can certainly cause cretinism (unnatural shortness or dwarfism) or interrupted growth in children. This condition is usually obvious, and is often accompanied by the presence of other symptoms such as a goiter. In North America, hypothyroidism in children is almost always recognized early and treated and corrected by a pediatrician or endocrinologist through prescribed thyroid supplements. In fact, any child born in the United States or Canada is routinely screened for thyroid disease by law. However, height in children, teens, and adults is usually an inherited trait. Adults who are shorter than average generally can't attribute their shortness to a thyroid condition. All kinds of factors contribute to growth and height: genetics, environment, nutrition, diet, activity, and exercise. For example, someone who grew up in an area where milk, vegetables, or other basic dietary requirements weren't available may indeed be shorter than average. Often, if immigrants or refugees from underdeveloped countries have their children in more developed parts of the world, the children will grow taller because of better diet and nutrition. See chapter 9 for more details.

MYTH: *All mentally handicapped people have a thyroid problem.*

FACT: Undetected and uncorrected hypothyroidism in infancy can definitely cause mental retardation. In fact, prior to the introduction of routine screening for thyroid disease in newborns, congenital hypothyroidism was considered a major cause of retardation. (It still is in some countries.) For the last 15 years, however, all infants born in developed countries have been screened for hypothyroidism. In general, all kinds of factors can cause mental retardation: alcohol or certain drugs ingested during pregnancy, premature births, viruses, or high fever in infancy. The list goes on and on. It's a mistake, though, to assume automatically that someone is mentally handicapped because of a thyroid condition. Only a very small percentage of mentally handicapped adults can trace their conditions to a thyroid malfunction, and statistically only one in about 4,000 newborns are hypothyroid. See chapter 9 for more details.

MYTH: *Eating kelp improves thyroid function.*

MYTH: Kelp is simply seaweed and, like other seafood, has a high concentration of iodine. However, kelp is not a substitute for thyroid hormone and should never be taken as a substitute. The iodized salt contained in most food provides more than enough iodine for your body. Taking kelp can cause your body to overdose on iodine, which can interfere with thyroid function tests or lead to hyperthyroidism or a goiter. See chapter 13 for more information on nutrition and thyroid.

Tracing Thyroid Disease in Your Family

Sometimes truth really is stranger than fiction. For example, dyslexia, prematurely gray hair, hair loss, left-handedness, and *vitiligo*, a skin condition that results in patches of pigmentation loss (this is the condition Michael Jackson attributes to his "bleached skin" appearance) are statistically linked to thyroid disorders. Although all of these conditions are physically harmless, the presence of these inherited traits can point to long family histories of thyroid disease. In these times of rising health care costs, being aware of your family's medical history can often save hundreds if not thousands of dollars in diagnostic tests, treatment, and prescriptions.

Tracing thyroid disease in the family is also important if you are planning a family or already have children. If you're pregnant, trying to get pregnant, or unable to get pregnant, it's important that your doctor is aware of your family's thyroid history. If you are prone to thyroid disorders, you're more vulnerable to them when you're pregnant; and as discussed above, an infertility problem is *sometimes* linked to a thyroid disorder. (Pregnancy and thyroid are covered in detail in chapter 7.)

If you already have children and you know your family has a history of thyroid disorders, you can alert them to that fact when they're older (particularly daughters, since thyroid disorders occur more frequently in women) and encourage regular testing of thyroid levels in their late teens and adulthood. You can also alert your children's doctors to your family's thyroid history. Again, the point is to avoid unnecessary health costs and problems that can arise through misdiagnosis of either specific thyroid disorders or related disorders.

Statistically, dyslexia occurs more frequently in families where someone has been diagnosed with hypothyroidism, hyperthyroidism, or Hashimoto's disease (see chapter 3) than in families with a history of normal thyroid function. It's important to note, though, that the dyslexia itself is not caused by a thyroid problem. Usually, thyroid disorders strike the females in the family, while dyslexia strikes the males.

Dyslexia is a *correctable* learning disability characterized by a number of things: delays in physical or speech development, poor spelling or handwriting, stuttering, right-left confusion, and reversal of numbers or letters. Although dyslexic children may have difficulty reading and perform poorly in the academic arena, they are usually very bright and often gifted in terms of athletics, art, and music. Dyslexic children or adults are often left-handed or ambidextrous.

If there are children in your family who show signs of dyslexia, and if your family has a history of thyroid problems, get the child's school to suggest some counselors who specialize in learning disabilities. If you come from a family with a history of thyroid disorders and had similar difficulties as a child, or still confuse right and left or reverse letters, you may well be an "undiagnosed" dyslexic. Dyslexia is not a physically unhealthy condition in any way and is treatable with the appropriate tutoring.

Turning gray prematurely (that is, before 30) is a seemingly trivial family trait. It is a statistical fact, however, that premature gray occurs far more frequently in people with thyroid disorders than in people with normal thyroid function. Therefore, by tracing the genetic pattern of premature gray hair in your family, you can also trace inherited thyroid disease. Patchy hair loss is another clue that thyroid disease may run in the family.

Here's how it works: If, for example, you, your mother, your grandmother, and your great-grandmother all turned gray by age 25, you might suspect that thyroid disease probably runs in the family as well. You could then alert your doctor and request that he or she check your thyroid levels more regularly. That way, if you did develop a thyroid problem, you would avoid the possibility of a misdiagnosis or late diagnosis.

One 1992 study found that 70% of Graves' patients surveyed were found to be either left-handed or ambidextrous. So if there are several left-handed or ambidextrous people in your family, this may be a huge clue that Graves' disease looms large.

As for vitiligo, it is also a harmless condition characterized by patches of pigmentation loss (either white or pinkish patches) on the hands, arms, neck and face. If this condition runs in your family, alert your doctor that you are susceptible to thyroid problems. There are not many effective treatments for vitiligo, but there are some dermatological creams that may slow the pigment loss. Anyone with vitiligo should be under the care of a dermatologist. If no creams or medication help the condition, there are some hypoallergenic makeup bases that can be used to even out the skin tone and mask the condition.

Another way to trace a tendency toward thyroid disease is to track how many *other* forms of autoimmune diseases are in your family. Apparently people with other autoimmune diseases, such as lupus, rheumatoid arthritis, and diabetes (these are discussed in chapter 2), are up to 10 times more likely to develop autoimmune thyroid disease. Autoimmune disease also affects women at least five times more often than men, while many autoimmune diseases run in families.

Knowledge is power. That's why patients often feel powerless to control their own destinies and become dependent on their doctors. But the role of patient and physician is rapidly changing. We're living in an information age where much of what we know about good health and medicine comes through other sources—television, video, film, magazines, and the Internet. Knowing your family history is the first step to becoming more empowered as a patient, and hence an active participant in your own health care. The second step is understanding how various family diseases can affect you and your children.

If thyroid disease is part of your family legacy, or if you have a thyroid problem, you can alleviate a great deal of stress and depression by understanding more about your condition. There is usually more than one course of treatment available for most thyroid disorders, and you have a right to decide which path is the best for you—after all, it *is* your body. (For more information on how to deal with doctors more effectively, see chapter 10.)

Finally, it's important to understand that in most cases the thyroid malfunctions because of reasons beyond our control. Although it's possible that a low- or high-iodine diet can trigger a thyroid problem, it's unusual for this to happen in North America. For the most part, there's no particular diet, substance, or activity that can prevent or trigger a thyroid disorder. Most thyroid disorders occur because of our genetic makeup or are triggered by stress. Although a healthy lifestyle is always a factor in preventing disease, healthy, active people develop thyroid disorders just as easily as those who are less vigorous. The key is understanding the disorder once it develops, and getting it under control as soon as possible.

Over and Under:
Hyperthyroidism and Hypothyroidism

Chances are that anyone diagnosed or treated for a thyroid disorder experiences symptoms of either an underactive or overactive thyroid gland. Depending on the severity of an individual's disorder, these symptoms can range from mild to severe. The term for an underactive thyroid gland is *hypothyroidism* (*hypo* means "too little"). The term *hyperthyroidism* (*hyper* means "too much") describes an overactive thyroid gland. The sole purpose of the thyroid gland is to manufacture the thyroid hormones thyroxine and triiodothyronine (detailed in the previous chapter), which are essential for good health and control the body's metabolism and energy levels. A thyroid gland is underactive when it fails to manufacture enough of these hormones (referred to in the singular as *thyroid hormone*). When it manufactures too much, the gland becomes overactive.

In most cases overactive and underactive thyroid glands are *symptoms* of specific thyroid diseases; they are not the *cause* of a disorder, however. The best way to explain this is to imagine that you have a cold: Your throat is sore, your nose is stuffy, and your chest might feel congested. The sore throat and congestion are cold symptoms; the cold itself is caused by a virus. Similarly, hyperthyroidism and hypothyroidism are manifestations of thyroid disease; the thyroid disorders themselves are caused by particular malfunctions, some of which were outlined in chapter 1. Sometimes, to simplify explanations, doctors may choose only to tell patients that they are hyperthyroid or hypothyroid, sparing them the details of the actual malfunction that caused their overactive or underactive symptoms. It's not possible, however, to become hyperthyroid or hypothyroid spontaneously without there being the presence of a particular disorder.

Treatment for a specific thyroid disorder often results in hyper- or hypothyroidism. When this is the case, the under- or overactivity of the thyroid gland is a temporary side effect to the treatment, just as drowsiness can be a side effect of a particular cold medicine. This chapter explains what happens to your body when you are either hyper- or hypothyroid, and covers both the major causes of and treatments for these conditions.

Hyperthyroidism: Is it Hot in Here?

The Hyper-alphabet Soup

There are numerous physical symptoms that you can experience when you're hyperthyroid—so many, in fact, that I discuss them alphabetically. Hopefully, this can give you faster access to the information you may need *now!* The good news is that the vast majority of these symptoms disappear once your thyroid problem is treated.

Behavioral and emotional changes

You may experience a host of emotional symptoms, such as irritability, restlessness, sleeplessness, anxiety, depression, and sadness. See the sections "Emotional Effects of Hyperthyroidism" and "Hyperthyroidism and Psychiatric Misdiagnosis" for details.

Breast enlargement in men

The effects of hyperthyroidism on male reproduction is discussed more in chapter 8, but this condition is considered a classic sign of hyperthyroidism in men. Breast enlargement also occurs when men gain weight, and is caused by an overstimulation of estrogen which is manufactured by fat cells. At this point, whether there is a direct association between thyroid hormone and estrogen production remains unclear, but it may help to explain this symptom.

Diarrhea

Diarrhea is another sign, even if your diet is normal. Your digestion speeds up, which causes the diarrhea, and sometimes the buildup of thyroxine will prevent your small intestine from absorbing certain nutrients from food. If you suffered from chronic constipation prior to your thyroid problem, you may notice simple regularity without laxatives or fiber.

Easy bruising

Platelet disorders tend to be more common in people with either hyper or hypothyroidism because the number of your platelets—which help your blood to clot—are reduced. Aspirin or nonsteroidal anti-inflammatory drugs (NSAIDS), such as ibuprofen, can make the bruising worse. Your platelet function can be checked via a bleeding-time test. This disorder can exist without a thyroid problem, and may simply indicate that you're more prone to develop a thyroid problem down the road. However, this does not pose any danger to your health unless very large numbers of platelets are destroyed (this is a pretty rare occurrence). A watchful eye (yours and your doctor's) is the best approach for now.

Enlarged thyroid gland

As discussed in chapter 1, an enlarged thyroid gland is called a goiter, where your thyroid will enlarge and may swell out of your neck. A goiter (an overgrown thyroid gland) often develops because too much thyroid hormone causes the thyroid gland to enlarge. In extreme cases, a goiter can swell to the diameter of a midsize balloon, and may have been responsible for a few circus sideshows in the days prior to treatment. Goiters are also caused by iodine deficiency as well as hypothyroidism.

Eye problems

If Graves' disease, an autoimmune or self-attacking disorder, is the cause of your hyperthyroidism, you may also notice changes in your eyes; they can become irritated, itchy, watery, and bulgy, and sometimes double vision occurs. This is known as exophthalmos and is explained in detail in chapter 3.

Exhaustion

When the body is overworked, this can lead to exhaustion, which will affect your sleep patterns, energy levels, and general emotional well-being. See the separate section on behavioral and emotional changes for details.

Fingertips and fingernail changes

Many hyperthyroid people notice that they have swollen fingertips to the point where they look "clubbed." This is known as achropachy or clubbing. Nail growth also increases, while the nails become soft and easy to tear off. In addition, an alarming condition known as onycholysis can occur, where the fingernails become partially separated from the fingertips.

Hair changes

Hair often becomes softer and finer and may not be as easy to style as it once was. In some cases, you may notice hair loss and find clumps of it on your pillow, clothing, tub, or hairbrush. The appearance will be a general thinning of your hair, but once your thyroid is treated, hair should grow as it once did. To create less stress on the hair, avoid coloring or perms until the hair follicles are stronger. If you are self-conscious, get a wig and then take it to your hairdresser to style it as you normally wear your hair. You can also contact the American Hair Loss Council at 1-800-274-8717, also listed in the appendix.

Heat intolerance

A classic physical sign of hyperthyroidism is a particular intolerance to heat. Your body temperature rises, and normal temperatures feel too warm. As a result, you sweat far more than usual. The feeling is unpleasant because you feel isolated in your discomfort. Typically someone who is hyperthyroid is constantly wondering: Is it me, or is it *really* hot in here?

This single symptom is responsible for misdiagnosis of hyperthyroidism in women approaching menopause. Complaints of "feeling hot" are mistaken for "hot flashes," a classic menopausal symptom.

Heart palpitations

One of the first signs of hyperthyroidism is a rapid, forceful heartbeat. Increased levels of thyroxine released from the thyroid gland stimulate the heart to beat faster and harder. Initially, you won't notice an increase in your heart rate until it becomes severe. When your heartbeat is noticeably fast, and you're conscious of it beating in your chest, you experience what is called a palpitation. Generally, palpitations can occur from excessive exercise, sexual activity, alcohol or caffeine consumption, or smoking, and it is abnormal for a palpitation to occur when your body is inactive, not anxious, or not exposed to substances known to increase your heart rate. Yet hyperthyroid patients often experience palpitations when they're quietly reading, sleeping, or involved in other relaxing activities. Palpitations caused by an overactive thyroid gland, however, do not mean you have a serious heart condition. When your hyperthyroidism is treated, your heart resumes its normal rate.

Untreated palpitations caused by hyperthyroidism can lead to serious heart problems and can eventually cause heart failure. Normally, a hyperthyroid condition is caught in its early stages, long before any serious heart problem develops. In fact, permanent changes in the heart are unusual in patients with normal, healthy hearts unless hyperthyroidism is particularly severe and left untreated.

If you have normal thyroid function and take synthetic thyroid hormone when it's not prescribed (helping yourself to a friend's or relative's supply, for example), you'll mostly likely overwork your heart and put yourself unnecessarily at risk. This is why it's dangerous to misuse synthetic thyroid hormone and why it should never be used as a weight-control pill. In addition, women who use synthetic thyroid hormone as a weight-control pill can drastically and dangerously aggravate a weight-loss program or diet they may already be on.

As many as 15% of all hyperthyroid people experience atrial fibrillation, a common heart rhythm abnormality. This means that your heart may pause slightly, followed by bursts of pounding, rapid heartbeats. This may be only an occasional symptom, but it's not unusual for it to continue until the thyroid problem is treated.

Thyroid-related heart problems are treated with beta blockers that slow the heart down (discussed more in chapter 12), but there is a large percentage of thyroid patients misdiagnosed as cardiac patients for obvious reasons.

Infertility

Hyperthyroidism can interfere with a woman's ovulation cycle as well as a man's sperm cycle, causing temporary infertility. Once the thyroid problem is treated, however, fertility is restored.

An undiagnosed thyroid problem in early pregnancy can lead to miscarriage; repeated miscarriage is often considered a form of infertility. If this is a problem for you, *have your thyroid checked* to rule out an underlying thyroid problem.

Menstrual cycle changes

Hyperthyroid women will find that their periods are lighter and scantier, and they may even skip periods. This is why thyroid problems can affect fertility—because it interferes with ovulation and regular cycles. Once the thyroid problem is treated, cycles should return to normal. See chapter 7 for more details.

Muscle weakness

This is especially noticeable in the shoulders, hips, and thighs. Thigh muscles may, in fact, burn or feel soft when climbing stairs. Shoulder weakness is noticeable when you brush your hair or do upper arm movements for long periods of time. This may greatly exacerbate osteoporosis, discussed in chapter 7. Muscle weakness is partly due to an overworked, exhausted body, and will resolve once the thyroid problem is treated.

Paralysis

This is a rare symptom of Graves' disease (discussed in chapter 3), where you may find episodes of paralysis following exercise or after eating a lot of starch and sugars. This particularly affects people of Asian decent, but once the thyroid problem is brought under control, the paralysis resolves.

Sexual dysfunction

Both men and women can experience a decreased libido which, in men, can lead to temporary impotence. Sexual desire should be restored once you're treated.

Skin changes

Your skin may develop a fine, silky texture, while you may also notice patches of either pigmentation loss or tanning. People with Graves' disease also may notice thick or swollen skin over their shin bones. Also, see hives under the Hypo-alphabet.

Tremors

Trembling hands is one of the classic signs of hyperthyroidism. This symptom was dramatized in one of the first episodes of *Chicago Hope*, where an elderly surgeon, who was about to be ousted by the hospital board because of his hand tremors, was diagnosed in the nick of time by a younger surgeon who recognized the tremor as a sign of hyperthyroidism.

Weight loss

Sometimes the diarrhea, combined with heavy sweating, contributes to weight loss in spite of a healthy appetite. Women in particular find weight loss a unique bonus to a hyperthyroid condition, but it is this single hyperthyroid trait that causes a misunderstanding of thyroid and weight loss. Weight loss is usually limited to 10 to 20 pounds, and not all patients necessarily lose weight. Hyperthyroidism often causes excessive exhaustion, and some patients end up gaining weight because they become less active. Unfortunately, some women with normal thyroid function take synthetic thyroid hormone to induce weight loss. This is a big mistake and can cause heart trouble, along with a host of other unpleasant side effects.

The Emotional Effects of Hyperthyroidism

Normally, cells in the body use thyroid hormone to convert oxygen and calories into energy. When the body speeds up, however, there is almost too much energy. As a result, exhaustion can set in because the body simply can't store the excess energy. This is the paradox of hyperthyroidism: on one hand, bodily functions are speeding; on the other hand, mental and physical energy levels are literally exhausted. Consequently, hyperthyroid patients experience a range of emotional symptoms. Nervousness, restlessness, anxiety, irritability, sleeplessness (inability to sustain sleep for long periods of time) and insomnia (inability to fall asleep at all) are common problems. Basically, these are linked to a general fatigue caused by a very real physical exhaustion. A hyperthyroid person may exhibit some, all, or none of these characteristics; it depends on the individual.

Most hyperthyroid patients do experience loss of sleep, however. Under normal circumstances, the body slows down when it sleeps, which is why you usually feel refreshed when you wake up. But when you're hyperthyroid, the body continues to speed during sleep, and you often feel *more* tired when you wake up. This is another reason why irritability, anxiety, and general restlessness persist.

It is the emotional symptoms of hyperthyroidism that historically have caused the greatest trauma for thyroid patients. Again, each hyperthyroid patient is different and experiences different mixes of the classic hyperthyroid traits.

Hyperthyroidism and Psychiatric Misdiagnosis

Psychiatrists see so many thyroid patients referred to them as psychiatric patients, that thyroid function tests are now industry standards for most psychiatric referrals. In fact, one psychiatrist told me that thyroid patients are the most common misreferrals he gets in his practice.

When patients experience the exhaustion of hyperthyroidism and the natural anxiety that accompanies it but fail to notice or report other physical manifestations, such as a fast pulse or diarrhea, they are often misdiagnosed. Unfortunately, it is women in particular who suffer from continuous and classic thyroid misdiagnosis.

One reason is that thyroid disorders occur five to seven times more frequently in women (according to conservative estimates). Another reason is that hyperthyroid symptoms often imitate the symptoms of two psychiatric conditions known as major depression and manic depression. Less obvious reasons have to do with the sociological roles men and women play in the medical community. Too often, the drama of thyroid misdiagnosis has to do with the conditioning of traditionally male doctors and dependent female patients—a scenario that has only begun to shift in the last 20 years.

Major depression presents three main groups of symptoms. The first group has to do with depressed moods, which include irritability and sadness. The second group of symptoms involves a change in physical functions, including poor appetite, weight loss, sleeplessness, lack of energy, and a lack of sex drive. The third group deals with cognitive problems, in which anxiety is prevalent and events are interpreted or perceived oddly.

Hyperthyroid symptoms mimic manifestations in all three of these psychiatric groups. Until the mid-1970s, hyperthyroid women were diagnosed as hysterical, depressed, or emotionally unbalanced and were often referred to psychiatrists. As stress-related ailments became more prevalent in the 1980s and 1990s, hyperthyroid women were often told that they were under too much stress. Although stress-related exhaustion is a very real phenomenon in our time and can indeed cause anxiety, insomnia, and other problems, hyperthyroidism is still a prevalent and very real physical condition that is often overlooked. Chapter 10 discusses ways to become more conscious as a patient so you can make maximum use of your doctor's diagnostic skills. That's why reporting as many symptoms as you can is key. Hyperthyroid symptoms run in groups and usually are not isolated. Even subtle, physical changes can be noticed once you're made aware of them.

Finally, hyperthyroidism can sometimes cause euphoric mood swings, a characteristic of a psychiatric condition known as mania, which is present in manic depression. The good news is that times are definitely changing. There's a current movement in the psychiatric profession that is in favor of prescreening for thyroid problems when patients exhibit manic behavior. This will protect thyroid patients from being given antidepressants or other inappropriate drugs. Furthermore, when a psychiatrist suspects a thyroid condition and confirms it with a blood test, the psychiatrist will always consult an endocrinologist. At this point, the patient will probably be released into the endocrinologist's care.

It is possible for people to have both a thyroid condition and a psychiatric disorder, because both are common. In these cases, the psychiatric symptoms may result after a thyroid condition has been treated, or they may persist despite thyroid treatment. In short, someone with a thyroid condition is not necessarily exempt from a psychiatric illness.

What Causes Hyperthyroidism?

Although there can be several reasons why a thyroid gland would become overactive, in 80% of the cases the cause is from an autoimmune disorder known as Graves' disease. With an autoimmune disorder, the body, for reasons not yet known, turns against itself. In most advanced cases of Graves' disease, goiters develop, but with the sophistication and refinement of various blood tests, Graves' disease is often caught long before the thyroid noticeably enlarges. Autoimmune disorders and Graves' disease are discussed thoroughly in chapter 3.

A toxic multinodular goiter causes hyperthyroidism as well. Also known as Plummer's syndrome, this disorder is common in women over 60. A multi-nodular goiter is an enlarged thyroid gland that has noticeable lumps and bumps on it. The lumps somehow take on a thyroid life of their own; they become a sort of thyroid island, forming miniature thyroid hormone factories, so to speak. These lumps were described in chapter 1 as "wanna-be" thyroid glands, because they imitate the main gland and in time develop the ability to function independently. The problem is that the main gland continues making thyroid hormone, unaware that these lumps have separated themselves from it to become thyroid hormone entrepreneurs. Once the nodules make abnormally increased amounts of T_4, thyroid stimulating hormone (TSH) becomes suppressed, causing the main gland to quit making T_4. Sometimes a solitary toxic adenoma develops and causes hyperthyroidism. This is a benign growth that takes over all thyroid gland function. (See chapter 5 for further discussion.)

Hyperthyroidism also results from taking too much synthetic thyroid hormone. Synthetic thyroid hormone is either prescribed as a supplement when treating *hypo*thyroidism, or prescribed as replacement hormone when the thyroid is either surgically removed or deadened by radioactive iodine.

When is the thyroid gland surgically removed? Until the late 1960s, the preferred treatment for goiters (regardless of the cause) was surgical removal of the thyroid gland. Today a thyroidectomy is usually reserved for cases in which the thyroid gland has developed growths of some kind or become cancerous (thyroid cancer is explained in chapter 6).

When is radioactive iodine used? In general, it's used to shrink hyperthyroid goiters caused by Graves' disease. It's also used to treat a variety of thyroid diseases, including thyroid cancer. (For more details on radioactive iodine, see chapter 11.) Overdosing on thyroid supplement is very common in middle-aged and elderly patients who have had their thyroids removed or rendered inactive. The term *thyrotoxic,* which literally means "thyroid toxic," is often used in this case. This condition is easy to fix, however. Once the thyroid supplement dosage is stabilized, you become euthyroid (*eu* means "normal") again.

A typical thyrotoxic scenario is this: An elderly patient, who is seeing more than one doctor, receives more than one prescription for thyroid hormone replacement. How does this happen? Sometimes the doctors don't communicate with one another, and sometimes the patient doesn't inform the doctors that he or she is seeing more than one physician. The patient confuses the two prescriptions, fills them both, and accidentally doubles the medication.

Patients sometimes assume that an eight-month supply of pills—with roughly 20 repeats—means that they don't need to see their doctor for regular dosage monitoring. They end up filling the prescription all at once and use the same pills for over a decade. The reason this is dangerous is because our thyroxine requirements change as we age; we usually require less in later years. If, for example, a patient is taking 200 micrograms of thyroid hormone at age 60, by the time they're 70 years old, they may require only 100 micrograms. An older body metabolizes thyroid hormone differently, which means that smaller doses are more appropriate.

Another reason medication overdose occurs in later years is that doses prescribed 10 or 15 years ago were based on cruder hormone recipes and less sophisticated blood tests and monitoring systems. That's why it's important to get your dosage checked regularly. (Thyroid medication is discussed in detail in chapter 12.)

Testing for Hyperthyroidism

The signs of hyperthyroidism are often obvious, and a simple blood test called the TSH test confirms the diagnosis. TSH levels will read below normal when thyroid hormone levels are elevated. Sometimes, if a patient knows thyroid disease runs in the family, their doctors regularly check thyroid function via a blood test and can detect hyperthyroidism before any blatant symptoms occur. But when the symptoms of hyperthyroidism are not recognized, and the patient notices only subtle differences such as irritability or fatigue, misdiagnosis can also take place.

Usually, misdiagnosis means *no* diagnosis. This happens mainly because there may not be enough physical evidence present for a doctor to order the TSH test. However, it's highly unlikely that if a patient complained of a fast pulse, for example, a doctor would choose *not* to screen for hyperthyroidism. In short, the most difficult element in diagnosing (or ruling out) hyperthyroidism is getting your doctor to order a routine thyroid function test in the first place.

Once hyperthyroidism is diagnosed, other tests are given to measure the severity of your hyperthyroidism and to determine its cause. These additional tests can include blood tests that rule out an autoimmune disorder, radioactive iodine uptake tests, ultrasound, and fine needle aspiration.

The appropriate blood tests are those that check your *free* T_4 (FT_4 in LabSpeak) levels and your TSH. The term "free" refers to "unattached" thyroid hormone that travels in your bloodstream. Every hormone in our body tends to be "bound," or attached to a chemical protein in our blood. The bound hormone is inactive while the free hormone is active. That's why it's crucial to measure free, and hence, active hormone. If your doctor is ordering an older test, called a "total T_4" (TT_4 in LabSpeak), this should be combined with a T_3 resin uptake test, which also measures free T_3. For the record, the total T_4 tests are considered obsolete and have been replaced with free T_4 tests. Any doctor ordering a TT_4 on a blood requisition form should be questioned. In order to confirm or rule out an autoimmune disease such as Graves' disease or Hashimoto's disease (discussed in chapter 3), you will be tested for antithyroid antibodies or what's called thyroid-stimulating antibodies.

The only time thyroid hormone readings are difficult to interpret is if you're pregnant, on oral contraceptives, or if you're taking certain medications that may interfere with thyroid hormone readings.

Usually used in treating hyperthyroidism or thyroid cancer, radioactive iodine is used as a "tracer" in certain diagnostic tests. A common test used to measure both the cause and severity of your hyperthyroidism is the radioactive iodine uptake test. Here, you're given a minute dosage of radioactive iodine, which is then absorbed by your thyroid. The next day, when you return to the hospital, you'll be asked to sit in front of a huge, cameralike instrument. A conelike device is brought right up to your neck area. This machine, called a a scintillation, or counting probe, measures the amount of radioactive iodine absorbed by your thyroid by "counting" it.

If your hyperthyroidism is caused by an overproduction of thyroid hormone, your uptake, or absorption, of the radioactive iodine is high (usually more than 30% in 24 hours). If you are hyperthyroid but your uptake is low, your hyperthyroidism is probably caused by an overdose of thyroid hormone replacement or by some sort of inflammation in the thyroid. Radioactive iodine is discussed in more detail in chapter 11.

It's important to note that the thinking regarding radioactive iodine uptake tests has dramatically shifted since the first edition of this book. Many endocrinologists now believe that radioactive iodine uptake tests should be reserved only to determine why you have a goiter, why you have a lump on your thyroid gland, and whether you have a *cancerous* lump on your thyroid gland, and, sometimes, to find the cause of hyperthyroidism if you test negative for Graves' disease antibodies. Ordering this test to simply confirm hyperthyroidism or to simply see "how hyperthyroid you are" is considered a waste of time and money. If your T_4 readings are high, and/or your TSH readings are low, you're hyperthyroid. End of story.

Treatment for Hyperthyroidism

If your hyperthyroidism is caused by an overdose of thyroid supplement, the treatment is simply to adjust the dosage to an appropriate level. If your hyperthyroidism is caused by either a multinodular goiter or a solitary toxic adenoma, radioactive iodine, which shrinks the goiter, may be used to destroy the overactive parts of the thyroid gland; depending on the severity, a thyroidectomy may be performed. In either case, the goal of the two procedures is to stop your thyroid gland from functioning. To make sure the treatment works, your doctor will usually wait until you show signs of hypothyroidism before prescribing thyroid medication (hormone supplement). If you don't become hypothyroid, it means that you are euthyroid, or at a normal level, and may not even need to take any thyroid hormone supplement. In fact, after radioactive treatment, you can be euthyroid for years and then redevelop hyperthyroid symptoms. If you had surgery, some functioning thyroid tissue may have been left. Here, radioactive iodine would be used in addition to the surgery to deaden the remaining thyroid tissue. If you had radioactive iodine, a second treatment may be administered to deaden the surviving tissue.

Treatment for Graves' disease can take a variety of different courses, which include antithyroid drugs, radioactive iodine, and sometimes surgery. Chapter 3 discusses Graves' disease in detail and outlines the treatment thoroughly.

Hypothyroidism: I'm Cold, Tired, and Depressed

The Hypo-alphabet Soup

When your body slows down, there are equal but opposite symptoms to the hyperthyroid scenario. So again, I discuss these symptoms alphabetically so you can find the information you need faster. Also, these symptoms disappear once the thyroid problem is treated.

Cardiovascular changes

Hypothyroid people will have an unusually slow pulse (less than 70 beats per minute), and either too low or too high blood pressure.

More severe or prolonged hypothyroidism could raise your cholesterol levels as well, and this can aggravate coronary arteries. In a severe hypothyroid picture, the heart muscle fibers may weaken, which can lead to heart failure. This scenario is rare, however, and one would have to suffer from severe and obvious hypothyroid symptoms long before the heart would be at risk.

Cold intolerance

You may not be able to find a comfortable temperature, and may often wonder: why it's always so *freezing* in here? Hypothyroid people carry sweaters with them all the time to compensate for a continuous sensitivity to cold. You'll feel much more comfortable in hot, muggy weather, and may not even perspire at all in the heat. This is because your entire metabolic rate has slowed down as your body conserves heat by diverting blood away from your skin.

Depression and psychiatric misdiagnosis

Hypothyroidism is linked to psychiatric depression more frequently than hyperthyroidism. The physical symptoms associated with major depression (discussed in relation to hyperthyroidism) causes the psychiatric misdiagnosis. Sometimes psychiatrists find that hypothyroid patients can even exhibit certain behaviors linked to psychosis, such as paranoia or aural and visual hallucinations (hearing voices or seeing things that aren't there). Interestingly, roughly 15% of all patients suffering from depression are found to be hypothyroid. See chapter 12 for information on the effects of lithium on thyroid function.

Digestive changes and weight gain

Because your system is slowed down, you'll suffer from constipation, hardening of stools and bloating (which may cause bad breath), poor appetite as well as heartburn. The heartburn results because your food is not moving through the stomach as quickly, so acid and reflux (where semi-digested food comes up the esophagus) may occur.

Because the lack of thyroid hormone slows down your metabolism, you might gain weight, but because your appetite may decrease radically, your weight often stays the same. Hypothyroid patients can experience some or all of these symptoms, and sometimes, if the hypothyroidism is caught early enough, you may not be conscious of any of these symptoms until your doctor specifically asks you if you've noticed a particular change in your metabolism or energy. You'll need to adjust your eating habits to compensate, which is discussed more in chapter 13.

Enlarged thyroid gland

Your thyroid gland often enlarges because it's inflamed—

especially if you have Hashimoto's disease. But sometimes the destruction of the thyroid tissue can actually cause the thyroid gland to shrink. See the Hyper-alphabet for more details.

Fatigue and sleepiness

The most classic symptom of hypothyroidism is a distinct, lethargic tiredness or sluggishness, which causes you to feel unnaturally sleepy, and you want to sleep all the time, even though you slept well over 12 hours the night before. Your doctor may also notice very slow reflexes.

Fingernails

Fingernails in this case become brittle and develop lines and grooves to the point where nail polish becomes impossible.

Hair changes

When you're hypothyroid, hair may become thinner, dry and brittle, causing you to need lots of hair conditioner. Hair loss may also occur to the point where balding sets in. (See hair loss under the Hyper-alphabet for more details.) You will also lose body hair, such as eyebrows, leg and arm hair, as well as pubic hair.

High cholesterol

Hypothyroid people can easily develop high cholesterol, which can lead to a host of other problems, including heart disease. This should be controlled through diet until your thyroid problem comes under control. It's generally recommended to anyone with high cholesterol to be tested for hypothyroidism.

Hives

This tends to occur with thyroid patients who have either hyper- or hypothyroidism. Hives are harmless, red, itchy welts on the skin. Antihistamines usually take care of the problem.

Menstrual cycle changes

Menstrual periods become much heavier and more frequent than usual, and sometimes ovaries can stop producing an egg each month. If you're trying to have a child, this can make conception difficult. See chapter 7 for more details on menstrual cycle changes and infertility.

Milky discharge from breasts

Hypothyroidism may cause you to overproduce prolactin, which is the hormone responsible for milk production. Too much prolactin can also block estrogen production, which will also interfere with regular periods and ovulation. As a general rule, when you notice discharge coming out of your breast by itself, and you're not lactating or deliberately expressing your breasts, please get this checked out by a breast specialist or gynecologist, who should do a thorough breast exam to rule out other breast conditions. For more information, consult my book *The Breast Sourcebook*.

Muscles

Common complaints from hypothyroid people are muscular aches and cramps (which may contribute to crampier periods). In fact, many people believe they are experiencing arthritic symptoms when, in fact, this condition completely clears up once hypothyroidism is treated. However, the aching can be severe enough to wake you up at night. Muscle coordination is also a problem, and you may feel "clutzy" all the time and find it hard to carry out simple motor tasks.

Numbness

This is combined with the sensation of pins and needles, as well as a tendency to develop *carpal tunnel syndrome,* characterized by tingling and numbness in the hands. In this case, it's caused by compression on nerves in the wrist due to water retention and bloating. This condition also plagues pregnant women, who suffer from water retention, too. Carpal tunnel syndrome is also a repetitive strain injury and can be aggravated by keyboarding, for example. This condition should go away once your hypothyroidism is treated. More on this in chapter 3.

Skin changes

Skin may feel dry and coarse to the point where it flakes like powder when you scratch it. Cracked skin will also become the norm on your elbows and kneecaps. Your skin will also sport a yellowish hue as the hypothyroidism worsens. The yellow comes from a buildup of carotene, a substance in our diet that normally gets converted into vitamin A, but a process that slows down due to hypothyroidism. Because your body is conserving heat and diverting blood away from your skin, you'll look pale and washed out.

Other symptoms more obvious to a physician would be the presence of a condition known as myxedema, the thickening of the skin and underlying tissues. Myxedema is characterized by a puffiness around the eyes and face, and can even involve the tongue, which also enlarges. See the section on easy bruising in the Hyper-alphabet.

Stunted growth in children

The classic scenario is wondering why your 12-year-old son still looks like he's only nine-years old. So you take him to the doctor, and find out that his thyroid petered out, which is why he's stopped growing! This completely reverses once treatment with thyroid hormone begins. See chapter 9 for more details about thyroid disease in children.

Poor memory and concentration

Hypothyroidism causes a "spacey" feeling, where you may find it difficult to remember things, or to concentrate at work. This is especially scary for seniors, who may feel as though dementia is setting in. In fact, one of the most common causes of so-called senility is undiagnosed hypothyroidism. (So before you shout "Alzheimer's," get a thyroid function test for the loved one you suspect is "losing it.")

Voice changes

If your thyroid is enlarged, it may affect your vocal chords, causing your voice to sound hoarse or husky.

The Causes of Hypothyroidism

Hypothyroidism is often caused by an autoimmune disorder known as Hashimoto's disease, an inflammation of the thyroid gland. It occurs spontaneously or develops in conjunction with Graves' disease. Striking both younger and older women, Hashimoto's disease is caused by abnormal blood antibodies and white blood cells attacking and damaging thyroid cells. The insufficient number of thyroid cells leaves the Hashimoto's patient hypothyroid. In most cases a goiter develops because of the inflammation, but sometimes the thyroid gland can actually shrink. Hashimoto's disease is discussed more thoroughly in chapter 3.

Ironically, the treatment for a hyperthyroid condition often causes hypothyroidism. If a person with Graves' disease is treated with radioactive iodine, the thyroid gland is usually rendered inactive. Hypothyroidism will then naturally set in unless a thyroid supplement is prescribed. Similarly, if much of the gland is surgically removed, the absence of a sufficient remnant of the thyroid gland will immediately cause hypothyroidism until a supplement is prescribed.

Sometimes, for the purposes of accurate tests or treatment, your doctor may deliberately induce hypothyroidism. For example, if your thyroid gland was totally removed because of cancer, it may be necessary to undergo a scan later. In order for the scan to work, no synthetic hormone can be present in the body. Hence, hypothyroidism occurs. Or, if you were treated for Graves' disease with radioactive iodine, your doctor will wait until you show hypothyroid symptoms before putting you on thyroid hormone supplement, as explained earlier in this chapter.

When hypothyroidism is deliberate, your doctor will prepare you for the symptoms and may suggest dietary changes to ease the symptoms. Laxatives may be prescribed for constipation, a more protein-rich diet may be recommended to combat low energy levels, and skin creams and moisturizers may be needed for dryness. You may be warned to dress warmly because of the intolerance to cold that hypothyroidism causes.

Sometimes a baby is born with no thyroid gland. This is called congenital hypothyroidism and can lead to some serious problems. Today all newborn babies are screened for this condition through a heelpad blood spot test. If this condition is found to be present, the baby is immediately put on thyroid supplement and usually develops normally.

In addition, after childbirth as many as 10% of new mothers experience postpartum hypothyroidism, which is often shrugged off as postpartum depression, or postpartum "blues." Here, the thyroid gland can become inflamed after delivery and hypothyroidism results. This is often a temporary condition. (Chapter 7 discusses postpartum hypothyroidism in more detail.)

Finally, if the pituitary gland is affected by illness, hypothyroidism can set in. As chapter 1 informed you, this is because the pituitary gland regulates thyroid hormone production in the body, and the thyroid is very sensitive to it.

Testing and Treatment for Hypothyroidism

Twenty-five to 50% of all people who have received external radiation therapy to the head and neck area for cancers such as Hodgkin's disease, for example, tend to develop hypothyroidism within five years after their treatment. It's recommended that this group has an annual TSH test.

Again, it's getting your doctor to order the right blood test that's the hardest part of diagnosing hypothyroidism. It's far simpler, however, to test for and treat hypothyroidism than hyperthyroidism. A TSH blood test can determine low levels of thyroid hormone as the result of even minimal reductions in thyroid hormone production. Another blood test can also detect the presence of antibodies in your bloodstream, which point to an autoimmune disorder. Because these tests are very sensitive, and depending on how high or low your TSH levels are, your doctor can, with the help of a more thorough physical exam, determine both the severity and the cause of the hypothyroidism.

Treatment is simple. You will probably be put on synthetic thyroid hormone replacement for life. Normal dosages range between 100 and 150 micrograms. Finding the right dosage can sometimes be tricky; you may end up hyperthyroid from taking too high a dosage, or stay hypothyroid from taking too low a dosage. Usually, it takes over a month to determine whether the dosage is correct, and blood tests are taken at various intervals to check your hormone levels. Dosages are easily altered and adjusted accordingly by your doctor. Yet with the refined supplements and precise dosing available in this day and age, dosages are close to exact. Chapter 12 discusses thyroid medication in more detail.

Borderline Hypothyroidism: Nipping It In the Bud

The medical term for this is *subclinical hypothyroidism,* which refers to hypothyroidism that hasn't progressed very far and is still asymptomatic. On a blood test, your T_4 (or thyroid hormone) readings would be very close to normal, but your TSH readings would be high. Right now, there is much discussion in clinical circles about doing routine TSH testing in certain groups of people for subclinical hypothyroidism, which includes anyone with a family history of thyroid disease, women over 40, women after childbirth, and anyone over the age of 60. Because the TSH test is so simple and can be added to any blood lab package, this is an opportunity to catch and, hence, prevent hypothyroidism before symptoms develop.

As of this writing, the first rapid, one–step TSH test to check for hypothyroidism is now available to doctors' offices in the U.S. and Canada. Similar to a pregnancy test, but using serum instead of urine, ThyroCheck® has your TSH results in 10 minutes. The doctor will draw blood, spin it to serum, and place four drops in the test cassette window. If TSH is over 5mU/L, one line appears. The developers of ThyroCheck® anticipate that it will be a whole blood test soon, and may be available as a home test at drug stores within two to three years. The benefits are obvious. You would know that you're possibly hypothyroid and could immediately report to your doctor for further evaluation and treatment. If you are on thyroid medication you would be able to monitor your own health. You will soon be hearing of drug stores offering this test for general screening.

With its convenience, fast results, and low cost, this test could "revolutionize" thyroid testing globally, and I, for one, can't wait!

Things to Keep in Mind

Whether you're suffering from Graves' disease or Hashimoto's disease, hyperthyroidism and hypothyroidism are sister conditions. As discussed above, treatment for one may likely result in treatment for the other. The purpose of this chapter is to provide you with enough information about the physical and emotional manifestations of each condition to better equip you in relaying your symptoms to your doctor.

For example, if you've been noticeably lethargic and seem to have no appetite, why not take your own pulse? If it's slower than usual, you may indeed be hypothyroid. Or, if you've been restless, feeling anxiety-ridden, and losing weight, check your pulse. If it's faster than usual, hyperthyroidism may be the cause. The easiest way to take your pulse is to press your index finger to the area of your neck right below your ear lobe. You'll feel a throbbing, pulsing sensation. Then, looking at a watch or a clock with a second hand, count each pulsation for 15 seconds and stop. Take the number (usually anywhere from 10 to 25) and multiply it by 4 for your heart rate. Another quick way is to simply use one of those "Test Your Heart Rate" machines in your local shopping mall or grocery store. They usually cost a quarter.

Why take your pulse? The first reason is that knowing your pulse will help secure a faster and more accurate diagnosis of a thyroid problem. It's the *combination* of emotional and physical symptoms that points to a thyroid condition and prevents your doctor from misdiagnosing your symptoms. By reporting your pulse rate along with your emotional symptoms, you have some physical evidence to back up your claims.

The second reason is to help maintain a proper dosage of thyroid hormone in your system. *You* live in your body—your doctor doesn't—and if you suspect that you're on too high or too low a dosage of thyroxine, taking your own pulse may help to confirm it. Then you can let your doctor know your findings, and he or she will adjust the dosage accordingly.

When you decide to take your own pulse, it's wise to have an idea of what your normal heart rate is. The easiest way to access this information is to call your doctor and ask for your pulse rate from a previous exam. Try to get a reading from at least six months back. Take your pulse at home and compare the two readings. If your doctor previously recorded a heart rate of 80 beats per minute and your pulse is now 100 beats, you're obviously quite a bit higher. Or, if your doctor recorded 80 and you're now at 60, you're significantly lower. Five beats more or less is probably nothing to be alarmed about, but 10 beats off in either direction is a sign that something has changed in your body.

In a nutshell, any thyroid disorder means that the pituitary-thyroid regulating system has broken down. Once you're diagnosed, it's up to you to compensate and take over the regulating of thyroid hormone from your pituitary gland. If you only suspect a thyroid problem, you should have it confirmed or ruled out by your doctor before you take any further action.

Autoimmune Disorders

As explained earlier, hyperthyroidism and hypothyroidism are not diseases in and of themselves; they are consequences, or symptoms of a larger problem—mainly, a particular disease or malfunction of the thyroid gland. Often, patients are told simply that their thyroids are underactive or overactive. The doctor may then discuss what happens to the thyroid gland and your body as a result. You may be told why your heart beats too fast or too slow or why you're lethargic or exhausted, but you may not be told *why* the overactivity or underactivity occurs in the first place. In other words, what's the problem *behind* the problem?

In chapter 2, I revealed that 80% of all hyperthyroid cases are caused by an autoimmune disorder known as Graves' disease, and that hypothyroidism is frequently caused by another autoimmune disorder known as Hashimoto's disease. This chapter will explain what an autoimmune disorder is and discuss both Graves' disease and Hashimoto's disease in detail.

What Is an Autoimmune Disorder?

The word *autoimmune* means "self-attacking." But before you can really grasp this meaning, it's important to understand how your body normally fights off infection or disease.

Whenever an invading virus or cell is detected, your body produces specific "armies," called antibodies, which attack foreign intruders, called antigens. Antibodies are made from one type of white blood cell (called lymphocytes), and each antibody is designed for a specific virus, the way a key is designed for a specific lock. The antibody acts as the key while the antigen is the lock. For example, if you had contracted chicken pox as a child, you couldn't contract it again, because your body is now armed with the antibody that kills the chicken pox virus. That specific chicken pox antibody is useless, however, against all other viruses, such as the mumps or measles.

Our doctors often give us vaccines to prevent the development of a particular virus, such as polio. Vaccines work like this: The serum contains a small amount of a particular virus in a deadened, noncontagious form. Essentially, a vaccine shows your body a picture of the virus, the way the police put up "WANTED" posters of a particular fugitive. The vaccine serum stimulates your system to produce a specific antibody to combat the virus. Later, if you catch the virus, your body destroys it before it can do any damage. That's why you don't necessarily need to get chicken pox to be protected from it; you can be vaccinated against it instead. However, creating a vaccine is a painstaking, complicated process, and it can take years for scientists to develop vaccines to specific viruses. Polio struck at epidemic proportions throughout the 1940s and 1950s until a vaccine was discovered. Now there is a race going on to develop a vaccine to the HIV virus, which causes AIDS.

When you have an autoimmune disorder, your body loses the ability to distinguish foreign tissue from normal tissue. It confuses the two and perceives healthy organs as invading viruses. Your body then ends up attacking its own organs. Some doctors describe it as a sort of allergy, where your body is in fact allergic to itself. So in the same way that the body develops specific antibodies to fight specific infections, here the body develops specific antibodies, also known as autoantibodies, to *attack* specific organs. Many illnesses are in fact autoimmune disorders; Graves' disease and Hashimoto's disease are two of them.

Who Is Vulnerable to Autoimmune Disorders?

Anyone can develop an autoimmune disorder. Many autoimmune disorders are hereditary, and some disorders, although not hereditary, run strongly in families. This is referred to as a genetic tendency, or inherited predisposition.

There's a great deal of evidence, though, to suggest that stress is a major factor in triggering an autoimmune disorder. When you're under unusual or extreme stress, depression or exhaustion can set in, which weakens your immune system. What is labeled "unusual" or "extreme"? A death or a tragedy in the family is considered to be extremely stressful. Starting a new job, moving or relocating is also very stressful; getting married or having a baby is stressful. Generally, any major change in our routines—be it positive or negative—is stressful, but people cope with changes differently. What one person finds stressful may not bother another person at all. A recent study which surveyed Graves' patients and non-Graves' patients found that more Graves' disease patients were under stress. Experts believe that once the stressful period is over, and the weakened immune system bounces back to normal again, it may bounce back too aggressively and "attack" normal tissue. It's similar to what happens to a puppy when it's been cooped up all day—once "released" from its crate, it will go crazy and jump all over you, perhaps even biting you too hard, unaware of its own strength.

However, women who are either pregnant or have just given birth are particularly vulnerable to autoimmune disorders. During the first trimester, and in the first six months after delivery, the risk of an autoimmune disease is at an all-time high in a woman's life. During the first three months of pregnancy, the body is naturally more fatigued because it is busy providing nutrients (including iodine) for the growing fetus and adapting itself to the pregnancy in general. In fact, pregnant women are naturally iodine-deficient for this reason. Pregnant women are also immune-suppressed to avoid "rejecting" the fetal tissue. The immune system may then "rebound" to an aggressive state, causing an autoimmune thyroid disease. This is discussed more in chapters 4 and 7. After childbirth, the body is readjusting and undergoing more hormonal changes. This can cause the thyroid gland to become inflamed after childbirth and, as mentioned in the previous chapter, as many as 10% of postpartum women may then experience temporary hypothyroidism, or Hashimoto's disease.

Therefore, if thyroid disease runs in the family, Graves' disease or Hashimoto's disease is statistically more likely to strike during these times.

Graves' Disease (also called Diffuse Toxic Goiter)

The most common thyroid disease is Graves' disease. Named after Robert Graves, the 19th-century Irish physician who first recognized the condition, Graves' disease tends to affect younger and middle-aged women—usually between 20 and 40 years old and usually in their childbearing years. However, it's not unheard of for someone in their fifties or sixties to develop Graves' disease either.

Statistically, Graves' disease occurs 15 to 20 times more frequently in women than in men. Roughly 1% of the population has Graves' disease, including former U.S. president George Bush, the former First Lady Barbara Bush, their dog, and most recently, John F. Kennedy Jr. At one time, the Bushes' sharing of Graves' disease was considered a fantastic medical coincidence, but some data have suggested that there may be an infectious agent associated with Graves' disease at work. Some investigators wonder whether German measles (rubella) may also trigger autoimmune thyroid disease. This may explain why there seems to be *families* of Graves' patients. At a 1994 Graves' disease convention I attended, one endocrinologist related his experience of testing the Bushes for this infectious agent at their home (they tested positive). "Don't get blood on the carpet or

Barbara will *kill* you," George Bush apparently said, half-jokingly. To date, the infection theory is still just a theory. Much more study is required before there is a clear-cut answer.

Although there is strong evidence for the hereditary nature of Graves' disease, some doctors prefer to classify it as a disorder that "runs strongly in families." There's not much difference between the two claims. Something that is technically hereditary means that a specific gene has been linked to the disease. So far, doctors have not yet isolated a *specific* gene responsible for Graves' disease, but they do know that certain families have a definite genetic predisposition to the illness.

What happens in Graves' disease is that a specific, abnormal antibody is produced, called thyroid stimulating antibody (TSA). TSA

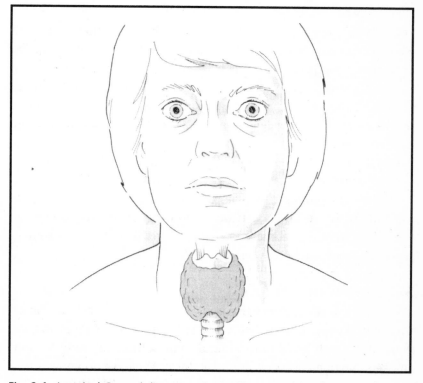

Fig. 3-1 A typical Graves' disease patient with a goiter and thyroid eye disease (TED).

Reprinted from *Nichts Gutes im Schilde Krankheiten der Schilddruse.* Copyright 1994, Georg Thieme Publishing.

stimulates the thyroid gland to overproduce thyroid hormone in vast quantity. Normally under control of the pituitary gland, the thyroid gland gets confused and is tricked into being controlled by the abnormal antibodies. The result is hyperthyroidism, and a goiter almost always develops. Yet sometimes the goiter is so slight that your doctor can't feel it.

Generally, the symptoms of Graves' disease are identical to the symptoms of hyperthyroidism, a condition *caused* by Graves' disease.

Thyroid Eye Disease (TED)

Although eye problems can occur with any hyperthyroid condition, people with Graves' disease tend to experience a peculiar strain of eye problems now known as thyroid eye disease, or in clinical circles as thyroid-associated ophthalmopathy (TAO). The prefix *ophthal* means "eyes," while *pathy* means "disease." It is this disease that lends itself to the expression "thyroid eyes"—bulging, watery eyes—a condition known as exophthalmos. This is a trait seen in Barbara Bush and was more pronounced in the late actor Marty Feldman, for example.

An eye problem associated with any type of hyperthyroidism is lid retraction. Here, the upper eyelids can retract slightly and expose more of the whites of the eyes. The lid retraction creates a rather dramatic "staring" look, an exaggerated expression. When the hyperthyroidism is corrected, the eyes often improve.

But the eye problems associated with Graves' disease are more severe. Many Graves' disease patients do experience thyroid eye disease. (Conservative estimates say roughly 10%, but several sources report figures as high as 90%!)

Smoke Gets into Your Eyes

Since the first edition of this book, one interesting fact has turned up about TED—it almost always attacks smokers with Graves' disease, while it is much less common (and some sources say rare) in non-smokers. No one knows exactly why this is. What we do know is that smokers are vulnerable to many more diseases and health problems than non-smokers. Clearly, TED is one of them. However, it is certainly not surprising that an environment where you're surrounded by your own or second-hand cigarette smoke would aggravate—or even help trigger—thyroid eye disease. In fact, one of the reasons non-smokers are so uncomfortable in smoke-filled rooms is because the smoke irritates their eyes, causing them to be watery, itchy, and red. Quitting smoking may help to ease some of your symptoms.

Symptoms of TED

The eye tissues are inflamed, causing the eyes to become painful, red, and watery, with a "gritty" feeling. Sensitivity to light is another common symptom. Some Graves' patients with eye problems are particularly sensitive to wind or sun. The covering of the eye is also inflamed and swollen. Meanwhile, the lids and tissues around the eyes are swollen with fluid, and the eyeballs tend to bulge out of their sockets. Because of eye muscle damage, the eyes can't move normally, resulting in blurred or double vision.

Other symptoms include discomfort when looking up or looking to the side. And, while some Graves' patients suffer from excessive watering of the eyes, many will also suffer from excessive dryness. In rare and extreme cases, the vision deteriorates because of too much pressure placed on the optic nerve.

During what's called the "hot phase," or the initial active phase of the disease, inflammation and swelling around and behind the eyes are common. This phase lasts about six months, followed by the "cold phase" where the inflammation subsides, and you notice more visual changes.

Generally, the changes to the eyes reach a "burnout" period within a two-year time frame and then stop. Sometimes the eyes get better on their own, but after the burnout period, the eyes usually remain changed but don't get any worse. The severity of the eye changes can be measured by an ophthalmologist (an eye disease specialist) with an instrument called an exophthalmometer. This instrument measures the degree to which the eyes have become bulgy.

The most common eye changes are bulginess and double vision. The impact of the eye disease also depends on age, sex, and occupation. There is evidence that middle-aged women and men suffer from eye problems more than younger men and women, while more stressful occupations seem to aggravate the eye problems.

Finding relief

Eye drops or "artificial tears" are recommended to relieve the irritation and inflammation. Wearing triangular-shaped, plastic prism lenses, which can be inserted inside your regular glasses, will help relieve double vision; or operations can be done at a later stage, which use similar techniques that correct squinting in childhood.

For deteriorating vision, there are a variety of approaches you need to discuss with a top eye surgeon. Treatments can include steroid medications, which can help reduce inflammation; decompression surgery; or external radiation therapy. The problem with steroids is that there are a host of side effects to contend with. If you have a temporary loss of vision, treatment will usually restore your vision, and only in very rare circumstances is vision loss permanent.

Recent studies indicate that thyroid eye disease is actually a separate disorder aggravated by certain autoimmune antibodies. Furthermore, thyroid eye disease is linked to Graves' disease only because of the reaction of circulating antibodies with proteins in both the thyroid cell and the eye muscle, which controls movement and puts pressure behind the eye muscle, causing it to be pushed forward. In other words, the attacking antibodies that the body produces in Graves' disease attack not only the cells of the thyroid gland but the cells of the eye muscles, too. The technical term for this is *cross-reactivity*. If this theory proves true, then thyroid eye disease can be treated by either removing or deadening the thyroid gland through surgery or radioactive iodine. Doing this also removes the TSAs that may potentially attack the eye muscle. It's possible, then, that thyroid eye disease may be preventable in the future.

Until the cross-reactivity theory is proven, thyroid eye disease is treated with hit-and-miss drugs and therapies. The treatment scenario goes something like this: The hyperthyroidism that results from Graves' disease is treated first (see the following section). In some cases, when the hyperthyroidism is treated the eyes tend to get better before burnout occurs, which supports the cross-reactivity theory.

Unfortunately, this doesn't always work, as in the case of Barbara Bush. The next step is then cobalt radiation therapy, or X-ray therapy. This procedure consists of X rays, CT scans, and a simulation procedure in which careful measurements are taken in order to aim the X rays properly; the X rays are targeted at the muscles at the back of the eyes, behind the lens, which can conceivably kill the cells causing the eye inflammation. The measurement is done using three laser light beams. About 80% of these treatments are successful, and the X-ray treatment isn't considered harmful. This treatment usually helps to restore lost vision. If the X-ray therapy doesn't work, there are operations that can be done to remove bone and expand the area behind the eye so swollen tissue can move into it. This procedure is known as orbital decompression. If the eye problems get worse no matter what is done to the thyroid gland or the eye area itself, drugs that inhibit the immune system are prescribed to prevent the optic nerve from being damaged. If the optic nerve is injured, blindness can set in, but only in the most severe and unlikely case would this happen!

The most disturbing eye problem is usually double vision, called diplopia. Some people cover one eye or instead of wearing prism lenses, which can provide some relief without medication or treatment. In some cases muscle surgery is necessary. Until the burnout period, most people with moderate eye problems just learn to live with double vision, since it rarely gets better. The eyes usually don't improve significantly, and in a small number of cases the eyes remain unchanged despite treatment for hyperthyroidism and a lapsed burnout period. There is now surgery available that can help restore your appearance under severe conditions. (The Mayo Clinic, for example, has reported some amazing results.) Discuss these options with your opthalmologist. There's no reason to live with a disfigured appearance.

Diagnosis and Treatment of Graves' Disease

Again, the signs of Graves' disease are often obvious: You may develop a goiter and display all the classic signs of hyperthyroidism.

Or you may develop thyroid eye disease symptoms, which are usually telltale signs of Graves' disease. When the signs are obvious, your doctor simply confirms the diagnosis with blood tests that check your thyroid blood levels and the presence of thyroid antibodies in the blood.

If you're not showing any blatant signs of hyperthyroidism but suspect Graves' disease because it runs in your family or you are experiencing more subtle symptoms, Graves' disease is again detected through blood tests that check thyroid function. As discussed previously, misdiagnosis is not uncommon, but today most physicians are more sophisticated in their diagnostic approach. If your thyroid function tests confirm hyperthyroidism, your doctor will then test for the presence of thyroid antibodies in your blood. Since Graves' disease is responsible for 80% of all hyperthyroid cases, most doctors routinely screen for it when hyperthyroidism is diagnosed.

There is no way to treat the root cause of Graves' disease—the autoimmune disorder itself. Therefore, treating Graves' disease involves treating the hyperthyroid symptoms. To treat hyperthyroidism, the thyroid gland is usually rendered inactive with antithyroid drugs or radioactive iodine, or removed through surgery.

To deaden the thyroid gland, radioactive iodine is the most common treatment. Radioactive iodine is simply iodine in a radioactive form. Since the thyroid naturally absorbs iodine to function, when the iodine is tainted or made radioactive, the malfunctioning thyroid gland greedily absorbs it and pretty well destroys itself in the process. (There is usually some residual thyroid function left.) Although this sounds rather drastic and gruesome, the procedure isn't dangerous and there are usually no side effects other than some minor swelling or irritation to the throat. The only time radioactive iodine isn't used is when patients are under the age of 20. As a precaution, children and young adults usually aren't exposed to radiation (although in more than 35 years of active use, radioactive iodine has not proved harmful yet). Given in capsule or liquid form, radioactive iodine effectively destroys the thyroid gland. (See chapter 11 for a more detailed discussion of radioactive iodine.) There is usually a waiting period after the radioactive iodine treatment is administered to see if the thyroid function has lowered. Usually the doctor will wait until you're hypothyroid before he or she prescribes thyroid replacement hormone to replace the output of a functioning thyroid. If your thyroid gland remains hyperthyroid after the first radioactive iodine treatment, a second dosage is administered. Sometimes three or more doses have to be used.

The second most common treatment is either a partial or total thyroidectomy, which is surgical removal of the thyroid gland. A thyroidectomy might be performed when there is a goiter, or when the patient is under 20 years old. This major surgery involves a general anesthetic and a postsurgical stay in the hospital of at least two days. There is a waiting period involved here as well. Sometimes small pieces of thyroid tissue are left behind, which could potentially reactivate Graves' disease. If this happens, radioactive iodine is used to kill off the remaining bits of tissue left behind. Again, when you become hypothyroid, thyroid replacement hormone is prescribed.

Doctors sometimes prefer to treat Graves' disease with antithyroid drugs. These drugs prevent the thyroid from manufacturing thyroid hormone. Then, as the production of hormone decreases, the hyperthyroidism disappears. Antithyroid drugs usually are used if patients are under 20 years old, but some doctors prefer to use them at any age. Sometimes patients themselves opt to try antithyroid drugs before more drastic measures are used. In general, antithyroid drugs are effective about 50% of the time, but some doctors report only a 30% success rate. These low "success rates" represent *remission* rates rather than *control* rates, so interpreting antithyroid statistics *correctly* is the key. Graves' disease, in virtually all patients, can be easily *controlled* with antithyroid medication. This means that the hyperthyroid symptoms caused by Graves' disease subside with antithyroid medication. However, when patients are taken off the drugs, only about 40% of them actually experience a true remission, while the remaining 60% will experience a recurrence of Graves' disease. Why even bother with antithyroid medication then? Many doctors feel that Graves' disease patients should have a chance at remission initially before more drastic therapies are used. It takes about six to eight weeks on the medication for the thyroid to resume normal function, but patients are kept on them for months or even years to determine if a true remission will occur. In the end, at least half the patients on antithyroid drugs wind up having either a thyroidectomy or radioactive iodine treatment. There is an upside to antithyroid drugs, however. Patients with eye problems see more improvement in their eyes while on antithyroid medication than they do with other forms of treatment. See chapter 12 for more details on antithyroid medication.

A final note on Graves' disease treatment. Some data suggests that radioactive iodine therapy doesn't work as well on Graves' patients first treated with antithyroid medication. If you're having radioactive iodine therapy while still on antithyroid medication, the current literature suggests higher doses of radioactive iodine if you've been *pretreated* with antithyroid medication. The general recommendation is to avoid antithyroid medication if a doctor knows for certain that you'll be having radioactive iodine therapy. Occasionally, after radioactive iodine treatment or surgery, there is just enough of the thyroid gland left to function normally on its own, meaning that thyroid replacement hormone is not necessary. This is not the norm, however. If you have Graves' disease, it's far more realistic to assume that after treatment you'll need to be put on thyroid replacement hormone for life.

Hashimoto's Disease

Not nearly as serious as Graves' disease, Hashimoto's disease is another common autoimmune disorder. It is a condition where the thyroid gland becomes inflamed. Clinically, inflammation of the thyroid gland is referred to as *thyroiditis*. Because of this, Hashimoto's disease is also called Hashimoto's thyroiditis.

It's important to note, however, that there are other forms of thyroiditis that are not autoimmune disorders; they are discussed in chapter 4. In medical circles, Hashimoto's disease is referred to as chronic lymphocytic thyroiditis because of the involvement of self-

attacking lymphocytes. The disease is named aft
the Japanese physician who first described the

Like Graves' disease, Hashimoto's disease i
most of the time it strikes women over 40 ye
many younger women have been diagnosed. St
women will likely develop Hashimoto's disease in
may also suffer from Hashimoto's disease but only abo. ... sixth
as often as women.

Hashimoto's disease is caused by abnormal blood antibodies and white blood cells attacking and damaging thyroid cells. Eventually, the constant attack destroys many of the thyroid cells. The absence of sufficient thyroid cells causes hypothyroidism. In most cases a goiter develops because of the inflammation, but sometimes the thyroid gland can actually shrink.

If you develop Hashimoto's disease, you probably won't notice *any* symptoms at all. Sometimes there's a mild pressure in the thyroid gland and sometimes fatigue can set in, but unless you're on the lookout for a thyroid disease, Hashimoto's disease can go undetected for years. Only when the thyroid cells are damaged to the point that the thyroid gland functions inadequately will you begin to experience the symptoms of hypothyroidism, described in chapter 2.

In rare instances, thyroid eye disease can set in as well. Again, the antibodies produced in Hashimoto's disease most likely aggravate the proteins in the eye muscle. Treating eye problems associated with Hashimoto's disease involves treating the initial hypothyroidism first. If the eye problems persist, the same treatment pattern outlined for Graves' disease follows.

Rarer still, some people with Hashimoto's disease experience hyperthyroidism as well as hypothyroidism. This "combo platter" happens because there are sometimes two forces of antibodies at work: those that attack and destroy the thyroid cells, and those that stimulate the gland to overproduce thyroxine, exactly like the antibodies involved with Graves' disease. This condition is coined Hashitoxicosis. Anyone suffering from this somewhat paradoxical condition would *first* experience all the symptoms of Graves' disease. Usually, after a few months, the antibodies attacking the thyroid cells over-

Graves'-like antibodies, and the hyperthyroidism cures it-
hen, as Hashimoto's disease progresses, you'd eventually end
hypothyroid unless replacement hormone was prescribed.

Diagnosis and Treatment of Hashimoto's Disease

The signs of Hashimoto's disease are not at all obvious. In the early stages, a goiter can develop as a result of the inflammation in the thyroid gland. The goiter is usually firm, but in rare cases it actually can be tender. The tenderness of the goiter can suggest Hashimoto's disease but it is usually suspected because of a sudden hypothyroidism or by the age of a hypothyroid patient, since it *is* common in women over 40. Hashimoto's disease is frequently misdiagnosed, however. Often, the hypothyroidism is attributed to age, particularly in women who are entering menopause.

Hashimoto's disease can be easily diagnosed through a blood test that detects high levels of antibodies in the blood. Another method of confirming a diagnosis is through a needle biopsy. A needle is inserted into the thyroid gland to remove some of its cells. The cells are then smeared onto a glass slide and examined under a microscope, which in the case of Hashimoto's disease would reveal abnormal white blood cells.

The treatment is simple: Thyroid replacement hormone is prescribed as soon as the diagnosis is made, even if there are no symptoms. There are three reasons why this is done. First, the synthetic hormone suppresses production of thyroid stimulating hormone (TSH) by the pituitary gland, which in turn shrinks any goiter that may have developed or is about to develop. Second, because Hashimoto's disease often progresses to the point where hypothyroidism sets in, the synthetic hormone nips the hypothyroidism in the bud and prevents the Hashimoto's disease patient from suffering the unpleasant symptoms of hypothyroidism. Finally, for some reason, synthetic thyroid hormone seems to interfere with the blood antibodies that are attacking the thyroid gland.

If you've developed a goiter as a result of Hashimoto's disease, the goiter usually persists unless thyroid hormone is prescribed.

Occasionally, though, the goiter shrinks on its own. On the average, it takes anywhere from 6 to 18 months for the goiter to shrink, and when it does, you'll most certainly be hypothyroid. However, a shrunken thyroid gland is often small from the beginning. (Remember, a goiter is simply an enlarged thyroid gland, so when the thyroid gland shrivels up, it no longer functions.) In rare instances, goiters can persist for years despite synthetic thyroxine.

Other Conditions Linked to Graves' Disease and Hashimoto's Disease

Graves' disease and Hashimoto's disease are associated with other conditions, just as Graves' disease is associated with thyroid eye disease. This section describes three conditions—anemia, arthritis, and diabetes—that are statistically more likely to occur in Graves' and Hashimoto's patients than in people who don't suffer from thyroid disease.

It's important to remember that if you have Graves' or Hashimoto's disease, it doesn't mean that you will definitely develop one of the related conditions described here. What it does mean is that if you're aware of some of these links, you'll be better prepared for the conditions should they develop down the road.

Anemia

When you're anemic, there's a decrease in the number of red blood cells carrying oxygen to various body tissues. Often, people who are hypothyroid are mildly anemic because of the body's tendency to slow down its functions. There are usually no specific symptoms associated with mild anemia, and it corrects itself when the hypothyroidism is treated.

A more serious type of anemia, called pernicious (meaning "serious") anemia, tends to occur in older people who either have or had

Graves' disease or Hashimoto's disease. Pernicious anemia is caused by a deficiency of Vitamin B_{12} (the vitamin responsible for producing red blood cells). When your thyroid is functioning normally, cells lining the stomach produce "intrinsic factor," which enables the body to absorb Vitamin B_{12} from food. Self-attacking antibodies to intrinsic factor occur in this disorder as an associated autoimmune disease genetically related to Graves' or Hashimoto's disease (like thyroid eye disease). The interference can prevent the body from absorbing the Vitamin B_{12} needed to manufacture sufficient quantities of red blood cells. When Vitamin B_{12} levels drop, anemia can set in.

Symptoms of pernicious anemia include numbness and tingling of the hands and feet (this happens because vitamin B_{12} also nourishes the nervous system), loss of balance, and weakness in the legs. Studies suggest that 5% of those diagnosed with Graves' disease and 10% of those diagnosed with Hashimoto's disease may develop pernicious anemia. However, because this type of anemia usually develops in patients over 60, younger patients with either Graves' or Hashimoto's are probably not at risk. But if you're 60 or older and have ever been diagnosed with Graves' or Hashimoto's disease, ask your doctor to specifically measure the vitamin B_{12} levels in your blood. If the levels are low or borderline, request an additional test known as the Schilling test, which can determine if you're having difficulty absorbing vitamin B_{12} from your food. If you do have pernicious anemia, it can be easily corrected with an intramuscular injection of Vitamin B_{12}. Usually the treatment is once a month, but it varies, depending upon the severity of the condition.

Arthritis

Some people with Graves' or Hashimoto's disease experience tendon and joint inflammation. Painful tendinitis and bursitis of the shoulder, for example, is reported in about 7% of Graves' and Hashimoto's disease patients, while it occurs in only about 1.7% of the general population.

In fact, rheumatoid arthritis (RA), a more serious disease, appears to be only slightly more common among thyroid patients than among the general population. Neverthless, RA can cause inflammation of many joints in the body, including knuckles, wrists, and elbows. Stiffness tends to be more severe in the morning. If you are either hyperthyroid or hypothyroid and have noticed this kind of pain or stiffness, ask your doctor to recommend appropriate medication for arthritic symptoms. Sometimes the pain and stiffness does improve when the thyroid condition is corrected.

Diabetes

There is an increased incidence of juvenile onset diabetes in families in which Graves' or Hashimoto's disease has been diagnosed. This means that if your grandmother had Graves' disease, you are statistically more likely to develop juvenile onset diabetes than someone who comes from a family with a history of normal thyroid function. This statistic holds true even if your predecessors *never* developed diabetes with their thyroid conditions. Similarly, if *you* have Graves' or Hashimoto's disease, your children and grandchildren are statistically more prone to develop juvenile onset diabetes. Juvenile onset diabetes begins in children or young adults and needs to be treated with insulin.

If you do happen to have both conditions, an overactive thyroid will often make the diabetes worse and more difficult to control with insulin. Once your thyroid condition is treated, though, you'll regain control over the diabetes.

Addison's Disease

This is when your adrenal glands fail to make cortisone and steroid hormones——the adrenal products your body needs to function properly. This is rare among thyroid patients, but it tends to occur much more commonly with pernicious anemia, which does occur more commonly in thyroid patients. It's interesting to note that John F. Kennedy Jr., who suffers from Graves' disease, also suffers from Addison's disease (according to the press), a condition which his father, John F. Kennedy, suffered from as well.

Inflammatory Bowel Disease (IBS)

This is an umbrella term that comprises Crohn's disease as well as colitis. IBS is a miserable condition where the lower intestine becomes inflamed, causing abdominal cramping, pain, fever, and mucusy, bloody diarrhea. IBS occurs more often in thyroid disease patients and can generally be controlled through diet and medication. If you have IBS, ask to be referred to a gastroenterologist, or G.I. specialist, who is the best specialist to manage it.

Lupus

This is a frightening condition that imitates many other diseases. For years, lupus patients went undiagnosed, similar to many thyroid patients. This is an autoimmune condition that affects many body tissues, causing arthritic symptoms, skin rashes, kidney, lung, and heart problems. Lupus patients often test positive for antithyroid antibodies. Interestingly, lupus is rare among thyroid sufferers, even though lupus sufferers often have thyroid problems. If you know someone with lupus, a thyroid function test is a good idea, which would at least relieve some of the symptoms.

Carpal Tunnel Syndrome

This condition is more common in thyroid sufferers than in the general population, and is discussed briefly in chapter 2. Carpal tunnel syndrome refers to a type of "wrist syndrome" in which nerves in the wrist become compressed. Conditions that cause water retention (or edema), such as hypothyroidism, can contribute to nerve compression. When the nerves in the wrist are compressed, all feeling in your hand can be blocked. Symptoms include numbness, tingling, or burning pain in the middle and index fingers and thumb. In more severe cases, all of your fingers may be affected, and numbness can sometimes extend to the elbow. If you're pregnant and/or hypothyroid and perform occupational tasks that place you more at risk for carpal tunnel syndrome, there's a greater chance that you'll experience this problem. Just stay alert to the symptoms and report them to your doctor.

Myasthenia gravis

When I did one of my first radio talk shows about thyroid disease, a caller asked me if I knew anything about this condition. I thought perhaps she was mispronouncing "Graves' disease" and feebly confessed complete ignorance. So I looked it up, and guess what? It is a rare autoimmune disorder of the muscles that affects only about 30 people per million, but it's *10 times* more common in Graves' disease patients! Symptoms include muscle weakness, double vision, and difficulty swallowing—some symptoms of Graves' and thyroid eye disease. What a nightmare if you have both! So ask to be tested for myasthenia gravis if you have these symptoms; they may not be caused solely by Graves' disease.

Bipolar Disorder
(formerly called manic depression)

This is a psychiatric disease where people experience extreme mood swings from elated mania to down-in-the-dumps blues. Bipolar disorder is caused by an imbalance in the brain chemistry and is controlled with lithium, known to cause hypothyroidism (discussed in chapter 12). Studies show that one quarter to one half of all people with bipolar disorder also suffer from a thyroid problem. If you've been diagnosed with bipolar disorder, get a thyroid function test. The emotional symptoms listed in chapter 2 may simulate a psychiatric condition, when in fact you don't have one!

The one theme this book stresses again and again is information. In an increasingly complex world where health care is big business and accessibility to health care is not what it should be, you as a patient benefit from understanding your illness and how your illness can affect other parts of your body. In the case of arthritis and diabetes,

Graves' disease and Hashimoto's disease are only linked because they are autoimmune diseases with a genetic relationship.

Autoimmune disorders are tricky because they mean that the body has turned against itself. There is not yet a vaccine which can prevent this from happening. For now, Graves' disease and Hashimoto's disease are only treatable because the symptoms they produce—hyper- and hypothyroidism—are treatable. These two diseases are good examples of when you *can* treat the symptoms and not the cause. Many health care professionals believe that the kind of emotional stresses outlined earlier (stresses which are beyond our control) trigger an implosion of sorts that manifests in an autoimmune disorder of some kind.

If you come from a "thyroid family" as I do, in which disorders are pronounced, you can prevent this sort of thyroid implosion by requesting regular thyroid level tests every couple of years between the ages of 20 and 50. Graves' and Hashimoto's disease are often caught long before any symptoms occur, and this is truly the best scenario.

What is unique about Hashimoto's disease (including post-partum thyroiditis and in most cases, silent thyroiditis) is that it's the only form of thyroiditis that is definitely caused by an autoimmune disorder. (Post-partum thyroiditis and silent, although autoimmune in nature, are discussed in chapter 4.) However, there are several other kinds of thyroiditis that are not autoimmune. The next chapter explains the causes of other kinds of thyroiditis and outlines the treatments for these conditions.

THE THYROID SOURCEBOOK

Thyroiditis:
Inflammation of the Thyroid Gland

In the United States alone, roughly 12 million people are affected by thyroiditis. Just as tonsillitis refers to inflamed tonsils, thyroiditis refers to an inflamed thyroid gland. Depending on what kind of thyroiditis you have, a goiter and symptoms of hyperthyroidism or hypothyroidism can develop. The most common type of thyroiditis is Hashimoto's thyroiditis, an autoimmune disorder described in the previous chapter. This chapter will explain other kinds of thyroid inflammation in more detail and discusses the three common forms and the two uncommon forms thyroiditis can take.

We usually associate inflammation with infection, the way a blister or open sore becomes infected. But the best way to understand thyroiditis is to think of it in terms of a giant swollen gland. In the same way that our lymph nodes or salivary glands swell because of various viral infections, the thyroid, too, can swell. In fact, after Hashimoto's disease, the main cause of thyroiditis is viral infection.

Subacute Viral Thyroiditis— A Pain in the Neck!

Subacute viral thyroiditis is also known as de Quervain's thyroiditis, after the Swiss physician who first described it. This form of thyroiditis seems to be particularly prevalent in North America, although Hashimoto's disease is about 40 times more common. It's suspected that subacute (or "not-so-severe") viral thyroiditis is probably caused by one or more viruses. Although there is no final proof that this condition is viral in origin, several possible viruses have been implicated that are similar to the measles or mumps virus and certain common cold viruses. This kind of virus is not contagious, however.

The condition ranges from extremely mild to severe and runs its own course the way a normal flu virus does. Usually, nobody with a mild case of viral thyroiditis would bother to see a doctor, because they wouldn't notice any unusual symptoms other than perhaps a sore throat. But in more severe cases you can be extremely uncomfortable.

The illness usually imitates the flu. This means you'll be tired and have muscular aches and pains, a headache, and a fever. But as the illness progresses, your thyroid gland will actually swell or enlarge from the infection and become very tender. It will hurt to swallow, and you might actually feel stabs of pain in your neck. To make matters worse, you can also become hyperthyroid. When the gland gets inflamed, thyroid hormones leak out of the thyroid gland the way pus oozes out of a blister. Gross but true. Then, of course, your system has too much thyroxine in it, and you experience all the classic hyperthyroid symptoms outlined in chapter 2.

The good news is that viral thyroiditis is quite temporary, and even the more severe cases tend to run their course in about six weeks; however, it can be a miserable six weeks, particularly if you don't know what's wrong. Although the condition *can* take longer to clear up, it's very unusual for it to linger beyond six months.

People suffering from this—women more commonly than men—usually go to their doctors with complaints of a sore throat, and the diagnosis is missed. If you point out to the doctor exactly where the swelling and tenderness are coming from, the doctor generally figures it out, especially if you tell him that thyroid disease runs in your family. Often though, it is the hyperthyroid symptoms that bring a viral thyroiditis patient to the doctor.

Subacute viral thyroiditis is diagnosed in part through the process of elimination. Because your thyroid gland is tender, the doctor knows it can't be Graves' disease. Hashimoto's disease is often suspected because of the tenderness. A blood test can easily rule out Hashimoto's disease because in this instance there would be no antibodies present in your blood. In more severe instances where a goiter may be present, radioactive iodine uptake tests are given. With this kind of thyroiditis, the results of the test would be extremely low because the infected thyroid cells would be too sick to absorb the iodine. A normal range for the uptake would be 8 to 32% absorption; with viral thyroiditis, the uptake is less than 1%. But since the condition runs its course, uptake tests are probably excessive.

For mild cases the undramatic treatment is aspirin to alleviate the swelling and inflammation. If the hyperthyroidism is more severe, sometimes a beta blocker such as propanalol is given to quiet your heart. In more severe forms, cortisone analogs are given. Sometimes the inflammation causes temporary damage to the thyroid cells and hypothyroidism can set in. If this happens, a temporary dosage of the thyroid hormone replacement thyroxine is prescribed until the hypothyroidism corrects itself. Basically, as the infection clears up, the thyroid gland resumes its normal, healthy function.

Subacute Thyroiditis: Part 2

While in many cases subacute thyroiditis clears up on its own, damage to the thyroid gland can sometimes result in permanent hypothyroidism, which means that you'll need to be on thyroid hormone replacement for life.

Silent Thyroiditis

Silent thyroiditis is so named because it's tricky to diagnose. It runs a painless course but is otherwise similar to subacute viral thyroiditis. With this version, there are no symptoms or outward signs of inflammation, but mild hyperthyroidism still occurs for the same leakage reasons. There are never any eye complications with this condition.

In the case of silent thyroiditis, there is no evidence that a virus is involved. There are some who think this type of thyroiditis might be a short-lived autoimmune disorder, like a mini-Hashimoto's disease. Silent thyroiditis sufferers are usually women, and the condition is common in the postpartum period.

This kind of thyroiditis was not recognized until the 1970s and was probably mistaken for Graves' disease before then because of the hyperthyroidism. Again, the thyroiditis runs its course and the hyperthyroidism clears up. In the course of the diagnosis, a silent thyroiditis sufferer is usually given a radioactive iodine uptake test because the test that detects blood antibodies in Graves' disease comes out negative. The uptake test then reveals the real cause of the hyperthyroidism, and the treatment is usually identical to that of viral thyroiditis. Often, no treatment is necessary, and the condition clears up by itself. This is sometimes referred to as Spontaneously Resolving Hyperthyroidism.

Postpartum Thyroiditis

During pregnancy, you're extremely vulnerable to autoimmune diseases due to a pregnancy-induced immune deficiency. If you manage to avoid an autoimmune disorder during pregnancy, after delivery, your immune system sometimes rebounds into a "super immune" state, instead of its normal, prepregnancy "on the lookout" state, causing it to be more aggressive and attack normal tissue. Some women, who may be borderline thyroid disease sufferers, are especially susceptible to thyroid trouble *after* delivery. In this case, the thyroid condition is usually a short-lived, temporary condition causing the thyroid gland to become inflamed.

Postpartum thyroiditis is a general label referring to silent thyroiditis occurring after childbirth, which causes mild hyperthyroidism, and also to a short-lived Hashimoto's-type of thyroiditis, which causes mild hypothyroidism. Until quite recently, the mild hypothyroid and hyperthyroid symptoms were simply attributed to the symptoms of postpartum depression or the notorious "maternal blues" thought to be caused by the dramatic hormonal changes women experience after pregnancy. But recent studies indicate that as many as 10% of *all* pregnant women experience transient (short-lived) thyroid problems and subsequent mild forms of hyperthyroidism or hypothyroidism. This statistic does not account for the many women who develop Graves' disease either during or after pregnancy.

Postpartum thyroiditis probably occurs because there is an advancement of autoimmune processes during pregnancy, followed by a postpartum rebound. The immune system is therefore most likely at this point to develop an autoimmune disease. Usually, the silent thyroiditis or short-lived Hashimoto's thyroiditis lasts for only a few weeks. Women often don't even realize what's wrong with them, because the symptoms are mild and are usually associated with the natural fatigue that accompanies looking after a newborn.

Diagnosing Postpartum Thyroiditis

Today, it should be standard practice for all pregnant women in North America to have their thyroid glands tested after delivery if they're displaying symptoms of maternal blues, postpartum depression, or thyroid disease. Regardless of how you feel, request that your doctor perform a thyroid function test after you deliver preferably before you're discharged. This simple blood test will determine whether you're either over- or underproducing thyroid hormone. If your thyroid test is normal yet you still have symptoms of depression or maternal blues, you can rule out a physical cause for your symptoms.

These conditions clear up by themselves. Short-lived Hashimoto's thyroiditis is usually more common than silent thyroiditis after delivery, and in more severe cases, thyroxine is given temporarily to alleviate the hypothyroid symptoms. However, women who experience this sudden thyroid flare-up usually tend to reexperience it with each pregnancy. Obviously, women who do experience postpartum thyroiditis are predisposed to thyroid disorders and seem to be vulnerable in that particular area. Since it's not feasible to screen for this condition in advance, there's really no way to prevent it.

Treating Postpartum Thyroiditis

Most women will experience hypothyroid symptoms. In this case, you may be monitored and given no medication unless the symptoms are severe enough to warrant it. Medication is one, tiny thyroid replacement hormone pill that replaces or supplements the thyroid hormone your body naturally makes.

If your hyperthyroid symptoms are severe, you may be placed on an antithyroid drug known as propylthiouracil (PTU), medication that quiets down your thyroid until it corrects itself. Treatment for hyperthyroidism is discussed in chapter 2.

Regardless of whether you're given thyroid hormone or PTU, you can still breast-feed safely.

Two Good Questions about Postpartum Thyroiditis

You'll be hearing more about thyroid disorders and postpartum thyroiditis in the years to come. Here are the two questions that all postpartum women should know the answers to:

Q: *I was diagnosed with postpartum thyroiditis over six months ago, and my thyroid condition doesn't seem to be going away!*

A: You probably don't have postpartum thyroiditis but postpartum *thyroid disease.* All that means is that you have a permanent thyroid condition that has developed after delivery. Most permanent thyroid conditions take the form of either Graves' disease (causing hyperthyroidism) or Hashimoto's disease (causing hyperthyroidism) discussed in chapter 3.

Q: *I'm currently being treated for a postpartum thyroid condition, but I'm still suffering from extreme emotional symptoms that don't seem to be related.*

A: Then they're probably not. Remember, just because you have postpartum thyroiditis or a permanent thyroid condition doesn't mean you can't also develop maternal blues, postpartum depression, or another more permanent psychiatric problem. In addition to seeing an endocrinologist, you should be under the care of a psychiatrist, as well.

For more information on pregnancy, see chapter 7 or consult my book, *The Pregnancy Sourcebook*.

Acute Suppurative Thyroiditis

Also known as acute thyroiditis, acute suppurative thyroiditis is a rare condition, but when it does occur, it's usually seen in children. The term *suppurative* refers to the presence of bacteria. Here, the thyroid gland suffers a dramatic pus-forming bacterial infection similar to the one that causes boils. The thyroid gland becomes painful and inflamed, and a high fever and chills accompany the infection. Sometimes there is an abscess within the gland because of the pus. Usually, the tenderness to the thyroid gland is obvious, so it's easy to diagnose. Antibiotics, incision, and drainage are the treatment, so even if the bacterial infection is thought to originate in the throat, the antibiotics clear up the infection anyway. (See chapter 7 for more details.)

Riedel's Thyroiditis

Riedel's thyroiditis is the rarest form of thyroiditis. Here, the thyroid gland is somehow replaced by a sort of scar tissue. The thyroid will feel tender and become very hard, like wood. Hence, the term *ligneous* (meaning "woody") or *fibrous* (meaning "scar tissue") thyroiditis is used to describe this peculiar condition. Because the gland attaches itself here to overlying skin and deeper structures in the neck, your windpipe might feel constricted, and your vocal cords could be affected as well, but this shouldn't affect your breathing. Your voice might become husky, and swallowing would be difficult. The diagnosis for this disorder may involve a biopsy to detect or rule out cancer, and usually the only treatment is surgical removal of the front part of the gland itself. The cause is unknown, but luckily it is an extremely isolated condition that hardly ever occurs.

It's important to keep in mind that thyroiditis is not life threatening, simply aggravating and uncomfortable. Some forms miraculously cure themselves within a couple of months. Occasionally, thyroiditis sufferers may find that they develop goiters as a result of the inflammation, or experience hypothyroidism because of permanently damaged thyroid cells. This is not the usual scenario, but it does happen. In these cases, thyroxine is given to alleviate the hypothyroidism. As for treating the goiter itself, the procedure varies. Sometimes the goiter disappears on its own, sometimes thyroxine helps to shrink it.

Overall, thyroiditis is relatively mild compared to other thyroid illnesses. The next two chapters discuss far more serious conditions that involve the investigation of thyroid nodules and treatment for thyroid cancer.

Please Explain Thyroid Nodules

The word *nodule* literally means "knot" and refers to a lump that can vary from the size of a pea to the size of a golf ball. The word nodule is used because people panic when they hear "lump." Nodule, the more clinical term, has been introduced into the thyroid vocabulary by the medical community in an attempt to soften the blow. In a cancer-phobic society such as ours, saying the word lump to the average person is synonymous with shouting "FIRE!" in a crowded theater!

Nodules are fairly common. One in 15 women and one in 60 men have a thyroid nodule, which translates into approximately 5 to 7% of the population. Yet only a small proportion of these nodules will ever turn out to be thyroid cancer. In fact, thyroid cancer is diagnosed in only about 10% of all thyroid patients each year—that's about 25 in a million people. And when it is diagnosed, it is curable 95% of the time. So what does this mean? It means that nodules on the thyroid gland are usually not cancerous, but when they are, the cancer is almost always treated successfully. However, the most difficult process in investigating nodules is finding out whether they are benign (noncancerous) or malignant (cancerous).

Investigating a Single Nodule

Either you or your doctor can feel a single lump on or around the thyroid gland. The lump varies usually in firmness but is small, smooth, and painless. Because the nodule protrudes from the skin, people often notice the lump on their own, or their doctors notice the lump during a routine physical exam. When a doctor discovers the lump, he or she will want to investigate it immediately. That way, if it does happen to be malignant, treatment can begin as soon as possible. Therefore, if you discover the lump yourself, see your doctor right away.

Single thyroid nodules are usually found to be one of three things: a growth that contains fluid (called a cyst), a growth that contains lazy, abnormal cells (called a benign tumor or adenoma), and a growth that contains active abnormal cells (called an adeno-carcinoma). Each is discussed below.

Cysts

Cysts that contain fluid are always benign. A needle biopsy immediately and easily determines whether the lump has fluid or not. A needle biopsy means that the doctor will stick a long needle into the lump and draw out some of the fluid inside. The fluid is then sent for cellular examination. This procedure is about as uncomfortable as getting a flu shot or giving blood. However, when the lump is found not to be a cyst, it is the difference between lazy and active abnormal cells that makes a lump benign or malignant.

Adenoma

An adenoma involves glandular cells, which usually clump together in a harmless, benign lump. Since the thyroid is a gland, any benign tumor that develops on the thyroid is called an adenoma. When abnormal cells grow on the thyroid gland, they vary in activity. Sometimes the cells are like bumps on a log; they are lazy and inactive and are just "there" without a purpose. It is as though the cells develop and then lack the drive or capability to do anything else. They don't reproduce, they don't imitate other thyroid cells, and they don't interfere with normal thyroid function; they simply exist. These cells live in a clump and appear as a nodule on or around your thyroid. When they're investigated, they're considered benign (harmless), which means that the lump is noncancerous. This is an adenoma.

Adenocarcinoma

The word carcinoma refers to a malignant (cancerous) growth that involves the epithelial cells, which line the surface of our insides. When a tumor in a glandular area is malignant and stems from these epithelial cells, it's referred to as an adenocarcinoma.

When abnormal cells develop, they are often far more active and purposeful. They spend all of their time reproducing; or they may spend only half their time reproducing, and the other half assisting or mimicking normal thyroid cells. They also live in clumps and appear as a nodule on or around your thyroid gland. When these cells are investigated, they are discovered to be malignant, which means that the lump is cancerous. This is an adenocarcinoma.

It is these active, abnormal cells that pose a threat to the rest of your body. Given the opportunity, they will mass produce themselves and invade, or metastasize, other parts of the body. (The word *metastasis* means "invasion.") That's why it's important to nip these cells in the bud. Generally, the harder the lump is, the more likely it is to be malignant. A softer, fleshier lump tends to be benign.

Solitary Toxic Adenoma

There is another kind of benign growth known as a solitary toxic adenoma (also described in chapter 2). Here, either a clump of cells or a singular growth develops and takes over all thyroid gland function. The adenoma is toxic in this case because it causes hyperthyroidism. The adenoma hijacks the main gland and assumes full production of thyroid hormone. The pituitary gland, which regulates thyroid stimulating hormone (TSH) gets confused by the situation and turns off. What happens then is that there is no monitoring system in place and the adenoma makes too much thyroxine. This is common in middle-aged or elderly patients. A solitary toxic adenoma is a type of thyroid disorder and is not malignant. It's easily treated with thyroid hormone replacement, which deactivates the growth.

The Diagnosis

Management of thyroid nodules has changed considerably since the first edition of this book. That's because of a diagnostic procedure known as fine needle aspiration (FNA). If you walked into your doctor's office with a lump in your neck five years ago, you may have had the entire lump removed through a procedure known as excisional biopsy—a nasty little procedure that was used to diagnose my own thyroid cancer. You may have also been sent for an ultrasound to see if your lump was fluid-filled or solid, and then had an excisional biopsy. These procedures are rarely necessary today.

FNA, a 20-minute procedure, is basically considered the gold standard now for evaluating a thyroid nodule. It can be performed in a doctor's office and is as simple as drawing a blood sample. The skin around your lump is cleansed with antiseptic, and some doctors inject a local anesthetic into the site before performing FNA. Many patients don't want or need this, however. The needle (which is finer than the standard needles used to sample blood), needs to be inserted three to six times to obtain a good sample. It sucks out cells and/or fluid (fluid if it's a cyst), which is sent off to a pathologist who is then able to determine if the lump is benign or malignant. FNA is accurate four out of five times. If your lump is a cyst, this procedure can also drain the cyst and collapse it, taking care of the problem entirely. The benefits of FNA outweigh other diagnostic procedures because it's cheap, easy, fast, accurate, and places far less stress on *you*, the patient. Studies show that because of FNA, thyroid surgery has dropped by 50%. This means that many people can be spared "look-see surgery," which was once more frequent when cancer was suspected. The end result is that while the number of thyroid cancers haven't substantially increased (in North America anyway), only half as many people need to have thyroid cancer surgery.

If there's a question about the diagnosis, or your doctor wants to get a *structural* picture of what's going on, you might be referred for a thyroid scan, discussed under "Hot" vs. "Cold" Nodules).

Ultrasound may also be used to check structure, too, but this pretty much has been abandoned in thyroid nodule testing because of FNA. At one time, ultrasound was useful because it told doctors whether the lump was hollow (a sign of a cyst) or solid. But today, ordering an ultrasound to evaluate thyroid nodules wouldn't give much information. You may want to request FNA if it's not offered, or at least ask why it's not being offered (there may be a good reason). For example, many doctors aren't trained to do FNA, while smaller communities may not staff pathologists trained to read the samples obtained through FNA.

Other Types of Needle Biopsies

Something known as a core needle biopsy (or cutting needle biopsy) was the "parent" of FNA. In other words, if FNA is a Pentium computer, core needle biopsy is a 386. It still works, it stills runs Windows, it's just not as fast and efficient as FNA. A core needle biopsy will be done if FNA isn't available. This procedure is exactly the same, except a larger needle is used and a larger amount of thyroid tissue is obtained, which necessitates the use of a local anesthetic. Core needle biopsies are also done in a hospital on an outpatient basis and may cause a little more bleeding and bruising from the puncture site.

Preparing for Needle Biopsies: Before and After

Anytime you have either FNA or core needle biopsy, it's a good idea to avoid medications that prolong blood clotting, such as aspirin, ibuprofen, and so on. If you're on prescription medication, let your doctor know prior to the procedure. Being on medication doesn't mean you can't have this done; however, avoiding medication just reduces risks of bleeding. Once the procedure is done, the puncture site will be bandaged and you can go home. You may have some neck tenderness or mild swelling afterward, but you'll be fine in 24 hours. If you develop a fever or begin bleeding, get yourself to a doctor or emergency room quickly; this may be a sign of infection at the puncture site.

Lobectomy and Thyroidectomy

When the lump is located on or within the thyroid gland itself, and the doctor suspects the possibility of a malignancy, he or she will perform more serious surgery that requires you to be under a general anesthetic. Depending on the size of the lump and where it is positioned, you may need only part of the gland removed. This is called a lobectomy, or partial thyroidectomy (the thyroid gland is divided into two lobes). Often, a good portion of the thyroid gland is removed under these circumstances, or a total thyroidectomy (removal of the thyroid gland) is performed.

"Hot" versus "Cold" Nodules

A thyroid scan is often done instead of a blood test and prior to a biopsy. This is an imaging test that photographs the structure of your thyroid gland. The test also involves a tracer of radioactive iodine. The thyroid scan is a 24-hour test, and its purpose in this case is to check for suspicious nodules. Normally, your thyroid gland absorbs iodine to make thyroid hormone. But when your thyroid gland is abnormal, radioactive iodine is absorbed (see chapter 11 for more details). In essence, a radioactive iodine scan measures how abnormal your thyroid structure is.

First, you're given a tiny amount of radioactive iodine and then sent home. The next day (12 hours later) you return to the hospital, where an imager takes photographs of your thyroid gland, which has now had time to absorb the radioactive iodine. Your doctor can tell how suspicious the lumps are by how much iodine they've absorbed. A newer tracer called technetium is now widely used in many hospitals. You're given a tiny amount of technetium and wait only two hours for your scan. This is obviously a far more convenient tracer.

A "hot" nodule is a lump on the thyroid gland made up of functioning thyroid cells. Therefore, these lumps absorb the radioactive iodine eagerly because the cells inside are intelligent enough to recognize iodine. Chances are, if the nodule is functioning, or hot, it is not cancerous. In these cases the lump found is either one of the nodules making up a multinodular goiter (described below and in chapter 2) or is a solitary toxic adenoma (described above).

A "cold" nodule is made up of more primitive cells that lack the intelligence to recognize and hence absorb iodine. A cold nodule is therefore more suspicious and is more likely to be cancerous. However, only 10% of all cold nodules found turn out to be malignant. A cold nodule means simply that the cells making up the nodule are abnormal and primitive. But it is the activity of these primitive cells that has yet to be determined, and that can only be done through a biopsy. If your scan shows the presence of only hot nodules, your doctor will probably not bother to do a biopsy, because cancerous cells are never hot. If your scan shows the presence of either a cold nodule, or a mixture of hot and cold nodules (usually the case with a multinodular goiter), a biopsy is always done to investigate whether the cold nodules are malignant or benign. A cold nodule merely means that it is a suspicious nodule and is *not* cancerous. Only a biopsy can absolutely determine whether a cold nodule is cancerous.

Benign Thyroid Nodules

Your medical history, age, and sex often determine the likelihood of whether a tumor is found to be benign or malignant. Older people usually develop benign nodules as their bodies age; natural wear and tear has much to do with this. Similarly, if you're an adult woman, it's far more likely that your nodule is benign; adult women, as a rule, retain more water and have more fat on their bodies than men. This is because women need the extra fat to menstruate and bear children. As a result, benign lumps can often spring up, particularly around the breasts. Furthermore, older women are more likely to have benign tumors on their thyroids than younger women. In addition, if you come from a family with a history of Hashimoto's disease or multinodular goiters, your lump is also likely to be benign.

Another sign of a benign nodule is whether you're suffering from hypothyroidism or hyperthyroidism, or have in fact developed a goiter in addition to the nodule. If you show symptoms of either condition (or both, as is sometimes the case with Hashimoto's disease), your nodule is probably benign, and is most likely a by-product of a defined thyroid disorder of some kind. For example, hyperthyroidism is caused by toxic adenomas or multinodular goiters, or thyroiditis can sometimes cause lumps on the thyroid gland.

A lump is usually benign if you discover more than one, or if the rest of the thyroid gland itself is enlarged or irregular in some way. Benign lumps also tend to be fleshier and softer, and can sometimes shrink slightly in size from one examination to the next. In fact, when a doctor first examines a lump, he or she will usually do nothing at that point, and instead ask you to come back in a couple of weeks. That way, the doctor can see if the lump changes in size at all (which is often the case). If it shrinks slightly, it's almost always benign; if it grows, it's more suspicious.

Malignant Thyroid Nodules

Certain groups of people are more likely to discover malignant nodules than others. For example, children, adolescents, and males who have nodules on their thyroid glands are statistically more likely to learn that their nodules are malignant.

Younger people (18 to 25) don't usually sprout benign nodules "just like that"; there's usually a reason for the nodule's presence. Therefore, if a nodule is discovered in a younger person, the risk of its being malignant is greater.

Similarly, when a male develops a lump, it's more suspicious than when a female develops one. Males have less fat on their bodies, and again, nodules don't tend to sprout on leaner physiques.

Finally, if you've ever received X-ray therapy to the thyroid region in the past, you're more likely to develop malignant nodules. Believe it or not, in the 1940s and early 1950s, X rays were used to treat a variety of ailments such as acne, adenoids, and tonsillitis. This is discussed in detail in chapter 6.

Recognizing the Symptoms

Usually there are no symptoms at all with malignant thyroid nodules. You'll feel perfectly healthy and your thyroid will actually function normally. The gland itself will not experience any change in shape, size, or efficiency. In fact, the only symptom is the presence of the lump itself. A single lump is more suspicious than several lumps, and if the lump grows in size, it's more likely to be malignant than if it doesn't grow. Malignant lumps also tend to be "fixed," or attached to the tissues around it, but this is a late finding.

Sometimes adenocarcinomas on the thyroid gland are found in a secondary stage. This means that the cells have already spread (reproduced) beyond the thyroid gland to lymph nodes in your neck. For example, it's not unusual for a person with undiagnosed thyroid cancer to discover a hard, little lump below the ear, or even further around the back of the neck. (In my own case I discovered a hard lump just below my ear.) If this happens, it means that the malignant tumor has spread to other lymph nodes in your neck. Lymph nodes are like small POW camps located throughout your body. Their purpose is to capture unwanted viruses or foreign cells that continuously invade our system, and destroy them. This is what keeps our systems running smoothly and efficiently. For example, if you have a bad cold or flu, lymph nodes around your ears will swell as the cold virus moves through your system. When lymph nodes are swollen, it means they've been switched on, or activated, by the virus. The same thing occurs when cancerous cells invade. The lymph nodes store these cells and become activated as they try to kill off the foreign cells.

If you notice a single lump in your neck, it's quite possible that the lump can be traced to your thyroid. This would mean that you have thyroid cancer. However, it's very important to note that not all lumps in the neck indicate thyroid cancer. First, lumps in the neck are extremely common and are rarely cancerous. Second, if they are found to be cancerous, they can be traced to other kinds of cancers, not just thyroid! Make sure you get all neck lumps checked out by a doctor before you jump to *any* conclusions.

In a more extreme stage of thyroid cancer, you might notice difficulty in swallowing or hoarseness. This would mean that the cancer is growing and pressing on other parts of the throat or neck close to the thyroid gland. But this rarely happens. The cancer would have had to remain undiagnosed or untreated for a long time.

Multinodular Goiters

The good news is that when you have more than one lump on the thyroid gland, the lumps are usually benign. The term multinodular means "many nodules." As mentioned in chapter 1, in the case of a multinodular goiter lumps form on your thyroid gland, mimicking the gland, and in time learn to make T_3 and T_4—thyroid hormone—as well. The nodules are completely unaware of the pituitary gland, which by contrast is aware of the intruding nodules. As a warning to the thyroid gland, the pituitary gland shuts off TSH secretion, and the thyroid gland slows down production. However, the copycat nodules continue to produce uncontrolled quantities of hormone. The result is an enlarged thyroid gland and hyperthyroidism, known as a toxic multinodular goiter. At first, the goiter and the hyperthyroidism may suggest Graves' disease, but a doctor can usually feel that the goiter is lumpy. Multinodular goiters tend to occur in postmenopausal women, while Graves' disease flourishes in premenopausal women. In addition, thyroid eye disease does not occur with a toxic multinodular goiter. So the absence of certain symptoms, coupled with your age, is often a strong indicator of the cause of your goiter.

If a multinodular goiter is diagnosed, a thyroid biopsy is usually done to rule out the possibility of any malignant nodule. You may be given thyroid hormone replacement if the nodules are not overactive, which in theory should shrink the gland, hence the nodules. But often the multinodular goiter and the nodules will not shrink. Many studies are now showing that radioactive iodine therapy is a more effective way of shrinking *nontoxic* multinodular goiters (multinodular goiters that do *not* cause hyperthyroidism). In these cases, thyroid hormone replacement doesn't seem to work. If the goiter is out of control (for example, it may continue to enlarge to the point where your windpipe is compressed) and you don't respond to thyroid hormone replacement, your thyroid may need to be surgically removed, which would solve the problem. Afterward, you'd be put on thyroid hormone replacement permanently.

The Nodule Journey

The best way to explain the process of investigating a nodule is to imagine yourself on a train that stops frequently at various checkpoints. You board the train when you first discover "the lump," and the journey begins. The first stop is your doctor, who will feel the lump and the area surrounding it *very* carefully. Your doctor may find obvious signs of a viral infection causing swollen glands that look like lumps, or your doctor may find signs of thyroid disease—such as a goiter—and rule out cancer or further investigation of the nodule. At that point, you can get off the train or you may have to continue on to the next stop, which would be a specialist. A thyroid specialist or head and neck surgeon may examine you. If the specialist rules out further investigation of the nodule, you can get off the train. If further investigation is needed, you may have to ride to the next stop, which is testing (blood tests, needle biopsies, thyroid scans). If the results come up benign, you can get off the train. If a malignancy is found, you'll have to stay on the train and ride through various treatment checkpoints until the end of the line, which is successful treatment. And that's exactly what the next chapter is all about—treatment of malignant thyroid nodules, otherwise known as thyroid cancer.

When They Tell You It's Cancer

Cancer is an emotionally charged word, conjuring up terrible images and nightmares. But cancer is *not* a death sentence. Certain kinds of cancer are more treatable than others; however, when detected in early stages, many cancers respond well to treatment—even more notorious ones such as leukemia and breast cancer. Leukemia is now treatable more than 60% of the time; treatment for breast cancer has made fantastic headway.

Since the 1940s, thyroid cancer has been *completely* treatable 95% of the time. Thyroid cancer is a particularly lazy kind of cancer that grows slowly and takes a very long time to spread. In fact, you could conceivably walk around with undiagnosed thyroid cancer for a decade and still respond well to treatment. Also, radioactive iodine (discovered in the 1940s) can often eradicate thyroid cancer. In a way, radioactive iodine is frequently a miracle treatment for thyroid cancer.

About 10% of all thyroid patients are diagnosed with thyroid cancer, in which abnormal, primitive cells have developed on the thyroid gland and are actively reproducing. Unless these cells are re-moved or killed off somehow, they will eventually spread and invade (or metastasize) other parts of your body. When these invasions, or metastases, occur, they interfere with normal bodily functions. In the worst-case scenario, thyroid cancer could spread to the bones or lungs. (It might take 20 years, but it's possible.) If that were to happen, then yes—thyroid cancer could be fatal. But the truth is, more people die today in childbirth than from thyroid cancer. If you have the misfortune of developing cancer, the thyroid gland is, in a sense, the best place to get it, because it is the most curable form of cancer.

Thyroid cancer is usually caught in a primary or secondary stage. In a primary stage, a malignant nodule or lump is found on the thyroid gland; in a secondary stage, a malignant nodule is found in a nearby lymph node, which is traced to the thyroid gland. (Nodules are discussed in chapter 5. Before you continue on, make sure you've read it!) Therefore, in a secondary stage, the thyroid cancer has already spread beyond the thyroid gland. In my own case, my thyroid cancer was discovered in a secondary stage, which is generally about as severe as it gets for the average thyroid cancer patient.

Who is Vulnerable?

For the most part, the cause of thyroid cancer is unknown, or idiopathic. Age and sex, discussed in the previous chapter, often determine who is more likely to have thyroid cancer. But anyone who has had X-ray therapy in the past is particularly more likely to develop thyroid cancer than someone who hasn't.

X-ray Therapy

In the 1940s and 1950s, X-ray therapy was commonly used to treat infants with enlarged thymus glands (which were falsely believed to cause crib death) and children with enlarged adenoids and tonsils. X-ray therapy was also used to treat facial acne, birthmarks, whooping cough, and scalp ringworm, and was sometimes used as a means to improve hearing for the deaf. The practice of using X rays began in the 1920s, peaked in the 1940s and 1950s, and slowly petered out by the 1960s. The treatment involved using an X-ray machine (this is called external beam irradiation) or placing a radioactive material such as radium directly in or on the tissue to be treated. The immediate results were often promising. For example, acne improved while acne scarring was reduced, and some forms of deafness were improved. (Enlarged lymph tissue would sometimes block the inner ear and cause deafness; radiation was used to shrink the lymph tissue and improve hearing.)

However, the long-term consequences of X-ray treatment canceled out any short-term benefits. Unlike laser treatment, X-ray treatment couldn't be concentrated on one small area without irradiating surrounding areas. Since the thyroid gland is located in the center of the neck, X-rays beamed at the face, adenoids, tonsils, thymus gland, ears, or scalp were also targeting the thyroid gland. By the 1950s, doctors began to notice an increase in benign and malignant nodules on the thyroid glands of patients who had previously been treated with X rays. Then, by the late 1950s and early 1960s, it was found that many victims of the atomic bomb that fell on Hiroshima and Nagasaki were developing malignant tumors on their thyroid glands. When these reports came out, doctors concluded that radiation was the cause. X-ray treatments were then banned.

It's estimated that millions of people throughout North America, Europe, and the United Kingdom received these treatments. (In the United States alone, more than two million people alone are estimated.) Generally, nodules have been discovered anywhere from 10 to 60 years later in people who received X-ray therapy in the past. Usually, though, people are most vulnerable between the ages of 30 to 50. If you have received these treatments or suspect you may have (often, children were too young and naive to realize they were receiving X rays, or the treatment was given to infants), get your thyroid checked regularly—at least once a year, and tell your doctor *why* you want your thyroid examined. Also, if your childhood doctor is still alive, contact that doctor and find out where your old records are. When doctors retire, they often turn over their entire practice to younger doctors, who often keep old records. (Usually, records are kept anywhere from 25 to 50 years after patients have left.) If you can remember where you lived when you received X-ray treatments, contact the hospitals in that area and request your medical records. To request old records, contact the medical records department of the hospital, or ask for the medical records librarian on duty. You'll want to ask what kind of treatment you received and how much radiation was used on you. Sometimes, hospitals will take the initiative and contact you by mail to inform you that you received such treatments. If you are contacted, see your doctor and arrange to have your thyroid checked regularly.

Radioactive Fallout and Thyroid Cancer

Radioactive iodine is emitted whenever fallout from nuclear accidents, testing, and, of course, atomic bombs occurs. Most unfortunately, we are seeing a tremendous increase in childhood thyroid cancer in certain "hot" areas, such as parts of Russia, Balarus, and the Ukraine. These regions were exposed to fallout from the 1986 Chernobyl nuclear reactor accident, which released 40 million curies (a unit of measurement) of radioactive iodine into the atmosphere. That's a lot, considering Graves' disease patients receive 10 millicuries (1/100th of a curie) in treatment, and thyroid cancer patients receive 100 millicuries. Reports of high rates of thyroid cancer are also coming in from Hanford, Washington, where residents were exposed to nuclear testing from 1944 through the mid-1970s (the mid-to-late 1940s were particularly intense).

Anyone living downwind from the Nevada Test Site (residents in southwestern Utah, for example) between the years 1951 and 1962 are also vulnerable to thyroid cancer, but there are many areas, particularly in the United States, that have questioned their thyroid cancer incidence.

Other areas affected by fallout are the Marshall Islands in the South Pacific, as a result of atomic bomb testing at Bikini Atoll in 1954. Here, thyroid cancer occurs 100 times more frequently than in the general population. In the aftermath of a very long Cold War, more information is slowly becoming available about just how "hot" North America, Europe, and other parts of the world really are. The predictions are that thyroid cancer incidence will continue to rise in our lifetime, but we're seeing this trend with a variety of other cancers, too.

How radioactive iodine affects healthy children

A child's thyroid gland is more sensitive to radioactive iodine because the thyroid cells of a child grow more rapidly than those of an adult. The gland itself is smaller in size, and therefore gets a larger dose of radioactive fallout than an adult. Thyroid cancer in children is actually considered an epidemic in post-Chernobyl areas of the Ukraine and Russia. It's of great concern to many surgeons worldwide. The cancer in these children is usually treatable, but we're seeing much more aggressive cancers in Chernobyl children than in other populations. I discuss this in more detail in chapter 11, and provide numbers to call for donations.

Since we're not really certain just how radioactive any air is these days, it's important to stay alert to lumps and enlarged lymph nodes on your child's neck or body (and your own!). Don't ignore these lumps, and don't allow your physician to ignore them, either. With fine needle aspiration (see chapter 5), these lumps can be easily evaluated.

The Asia-California Phenomenon

Another group at risk for thyroid cancer is Asian women who have immigrated to California. Studies have only just begun, but researchers suspect this has something to do with nutritional factors and iodine. The theory is that, somehow, when these women changed from an iodine-deficient diet as young women or children to an iodine-rich diet as adults or older women, the change in iodine content triggers thyroid cancer. These women are being tracked through toenail clippings, which are apparently good markers for trace elements. I'll keep you updated on this in future editions.

Signs of Thyroid Cancer

While most malignant thyroid lumps are hard and painless, there are some signs that a lump may be malignant. For example, if your lump continues to enlarge while you're on thyroid hormone, this is a clue that it's cancerous; thyroid hormone usually shrinks benign lumps. If you notice pain in your neck tissues, jawbone, or ear, have difficulty swallowing food or liquids, wheeze or have hoarseness, this may indicate that the cancer is spreading beyond the thyroid gland.

Statistics

Some surgeons report interesting statistics regarding thyroid cancer. For example, when a man develops a thyroid nodule (which occurs more frequently in women), some doctors estimate it's more common for it to be thyroid cancer (estimates run as high as 50%). This doesn't mean that 50% of all thyroid patients are *men*! It means that if you asked all of the men on earth who have ever had a thyroid nodule to step forward, you'd discover that half of them had thyroid cancer, and the other half had a mixture of various other thyroid disorders. Therefore, thyroid problems in men are statistically more likely to be thyroid cancer. However, only one in ten thyroid cancer patients is male, and thyroid cancer is now considered the most common kind of cancer in women ages 18 to 50.

Types of Thyroid Cancer

Thyroid cancer is divided into two categories: differentiated and undifferentiated. These terms refer to the sophistication of the cancer cells. Differentiated cancer cells act and look like normal thyroid cells. In fact, they actually assist the other cells with routine functions, such as making thyroxine. Because these cells spend some of their time assisting the thyroid gland, they spend less time reproducing and therefore take a lot longer to metastasize to other parts of the body. Differentiated cancer is the most common form of thyroid cancer. The cancer is more specifically referred to as a papillary cancer or follicular cancer. Papillary and follicular refer to both the physical shape and personality of the cancer cells, as well as the behavior of the cells. In essence, if papillary is blond and passive, follicular is brunet and aggressive. In other words, follicular is a more dangerous or *active* kind of cancer. However, it's very common for the cancer cells to be a combination of papillary and follicular cells. This is called a papillary-follicular mix. When this is the case, the passive, more "reasonable" papillary cancer counteracts some of the aggressiveness of the follicular cancer. For this reason, this kind of cancer is extremely treatable and has an excellent survival rate. In fact, a papillary-follicular mix is the most common form of thyroid cancer. For women under 50 and men under 40, the cure rate is just about 100%. In the worst-case scenario, this cancer has only a 17% chance of recurrence and only a 1.7% death rate.

When thyroid cancer is purely papillary, it's obviously far less aggressive than a type that is purely follicular. But the survival rate for both is still excellent; for women under 50 and men under 40, it's almost 100%. Papillary and follicular cancers tend to occur in younger people anyway, that is, those under 40. Hürthle cell cancer, an even more aggressive form of follicular cancer, generally can occur in people over 60. But because it is differentiated, this cancer is also very treatable.

Undifferentiated cancer is made up of very primitive cells that spend all their time reproducing. This is a very rare but more severe form of thyroid cancer, called anaplastic cancer. Anaplastic cancer cells therefore spread faster because they contribute nothing to the thyroid gland; their existence is devoted solely to reproduction. This cancer is usually discovered in elderly patients and is almost never found in patients under 40. The fact that anaplastic cancer generally develops in elderly patients is fortunate, because it is usually not treatable and the survival rate is not good.

Even rarer is a kind of inherited thyroid cancer called medullary cancer. This involves a specific cell that "rents space" from your thyroid gland, which secretes a hormone called calcitonin. This cell is called a C cell and can actually be detected through a specific blood test that checks for calcitonin. (See chapter 1.) If medullary thyroid cancer runs in your family, you'd probably be alerted by other family members or a doctor familiar with your family history. Then, your blood would be checked for calcitonin about once a year. Medullary cancer is less severe than anaplastic cancer, but more serious than differentiated cancers. It is still quite treatable, though.

Recently, a University of Michigan doctor developed a breakthrough blood test that can detect a specific gene placing you at risk for medullary thyroid cancer, which affects only about 1,000 people in the U.S. annually (a tiny segment of the population). If you test positive for the medullary thyroid cancer gene, you would undergo what's called a *prophylactic thyroidectomy,* meaning a preventive thyroidectomy. This removes the risk of *ever* developing medullary thyroid cancer, which can spread and develop into more serious cancer.

Sometimes a lymphoma develops on the thyroid gland. Lymphomas are cancer cells that usually originate in the lymph nodes but in rare instances can develop on the thyroid gland itself. Lymphomas involve white blood cells that go astray and attack functioning organs. For the most part, the only time lymphomas are ever found on the thyroid gland is when the patient has Hashimoto's thyroiditis (see chapter 3). Very few people with Hashimoto's thyroiditis have ever developed lymphomas, however, and lymphomas are still quite treatable nevertheless.

Finally, the presence of cancer cells on your thyroid gland can mean that cancer originating elsewhere has spread to your thyroid gland. In this case the cancer would not be thyroid cancer at all but an invading cancer that comes from a different place in your body, such as a kidney or breast. If this were the case, the origin of this metastatic, or spreading, cancer would have been detected long before the cancer reached your thyroid gland.

The Diagnosis for Thyroid Cancer

Thyroid cancer is typically diagnosed from a hard, smooth, painless lump that is either right on your thyroid gland or somewhere on your neck. You notice the lump yourself and bring it to your doctor's attention, or your doctor notices it during a routine exam. Some doctors will want to reexamine the lump again after two to four weeks before they proceed with further testing because only a small proportion of such lumps on the thyroid gland or in the neck are malignant. The lumps are usually benign, and reexamining the lump after a couple of weeks will either confirm or alleviate suspicions. (The previous chapter describes in detail the characteristics of malignant and benign lumps.)

When a lump is suspicious, your doctor may refer you to a specialist at this point. If the lump is on the thyroid gland, you'll probably be referred to an endocrinologist, a doctor who specializes in glands and hormones (collectively known as the endocrine system). The endocrinologist will decide what tests need to be done: a needle biopsy, an ultrasound, or a thyroid scan. (Chapter 5 describes these tests in detail.)

If the lump is on your neck and *away* from your thyroid gland, you may be referred to either a head and neck surgeon or a plastic surgeon. Lumps on the neck have many possible causes; head and neck surgeons and plastic surgeons are far more experienced with deciphering normal lumps from abnormal lumps. A surgeon will most likely remove the lump and do a biopsy. (See the section on lumpectomy in chapter 5.) When the lump is located on or within the thyroid gland and cancer is suspected, the surgeon will go ahead and perform either a lobectomy or thyroidectomy, also discussed in chapter 5. Generally, a total thyroidectomy is recommended.

Regardless how your lump is removed, the biopsy determines whether the thyroid cancer is differentiated or undifferentiated. When that has been established, the specialist will tell you the results of the test and outline the treatment that lies ahead. Your family doctor also will be notified.

Thyroid cancer is usually treated through surgery and radioactive iodine and managed by an endocrinologist and/or a head and neck surgeon. Sometimes you see both specialists; sometimes you see only one. If an endocrinologist finds the cancer, he or she will consult with a head and neck surgeon before going forward with treatment, because surgery will be necessary. However, when a head and neck surgeon finds the cancer first, an endocrinologist is rarely consulted before treatment. If this is the case, it's a good idea to request a referral to an endocrinologist before treatment begins. You will eventually come to depend on an endocrinologist for balancing your thyroid hormone after surgery, so the earlier you establish a history with this specialist, the better off you are.

At some point after your cancer has been diagnosed, you'll need to get some answers directly from your specialist or doctor. The best thing to do is make a separate appointment with one of them and use the entire appointment time for a question-and-answer period. Write down all of your questions ahead of time, and tape record the answers so you can review them later by yourself or with a supportive friend. When we're anxious, we often don't hear correctly; we misconstrue facts and block out what we don't want to hear. That's why it's important to tape your doctor's answers. What should you ask? Questions will vary from person to person, but here are some general areas to get you started:

1. Request the doctor draw you a diagram of the neck and thyroid gland, and shade in where the cancer is situated or has spread.
2. Ask whether the cancer is differentiated or undifferentiated.
3. Find out how long the cancer has been growing, where it can spread, and what stage it's in.
4. Find out where you can go for more information, and whether the doctor can refer you to a social worker who specializes in working with cancer patients.

Treatment for Thyroid Cancer

The usual treatment scenario for thyroid cancer involves a combination of surgery and radioactive iodine therapy. Sometimes, when the cancer is in a secondary stage, you'll need radiation therapy; only if you had a rare, undifferentiated, or anaplastic form of thyroid cancer would you require chemotherapy. Thyroid cancer generally has a very low recurrence rate. For most age groups and with most forms of thyroid cancer, the cancer only comes back about 17% of the time.

Surgery

Regardless of what stage your cancer is in, surgery is almost always used as a form of treatment. Even if your cancer was detected from a lump on the thyroid gland, which means the cancer hasn't spread beyond your thyroid gland and is therefore in a primary stage, a total or near total thyroidectomy is still performed. "Why take chances?" is the philosophy here.

When thyroid cancer is detected from a lump in the neck, it means that your thyroid cancer is in a secondary stage. Here, the cancer has spread beyond your thyroid gland to the lymph nodes in your neck surrounding the gland. In this case you'll need to have your entire thyroid gland removed, as well as the surrounding lymph nodes. This is called a total thyroidectomy. The surgeon will also want to examine seemingly healthy lymph nodes farther into the neck to make sure there is no cancer present. To do this, he or she will take out a few lymph nodes and, while you're still in surgery, quickly examine the lymph nodes under a microscope to see if there are any thyroid cells present. If there are, it means that the cancer has spread a little farther into the neck, and the surgeon will remove all lymph tissue with thyroid cells. This is called a neck dissection. When it's purely papillary, the cancer tends to spread into the neck; follicular spreads into the lungs and bones. A papillary-follicular mix behaves like papillary and spreads into the neck.

Only in rarer forms of thyroid cancer is surgery not recommended. Surgery, however, is always the first stage of treatment for differentiated forms of thyroid cancer.

Total thyroidectomy versus partial thyroidectomy (or lobectomy) is an extremely controversial issue right now with thyroid surgeons and endocrinologists. Many surgeons take the "conservation" approach where they want to leave as much thyroid tissue intact as possible. This is all very noble, but according to the best studies and top surgeons, this is generally the *wrong* approach when thyroid cancer has been detected—even if it's small and localized. And, since there is a small chance that thyroid cancer can recur, or that a surgeon may not be able to see every cancerous tidbit, radioactive iodine therapy is usually advised to "finish the job." The only time lobectomy is acceptable is if you have a papillary cancer less than one centimeter in size, or a highly noninvasive follicular cancer. However, given the choice, it may be worth having a total thyroidectomy in these situations to absolutely minimize your risk of recurrence and prevent the scenario of a repeat thyroid surgery. (I know people who have been through this!)

Radioactive iodine therapy following a thyroidectomy is an important way to eradicate all thyroid tissue—and hence, potentially cancerous tissue. A radioactive scan is an important way to detect a *recurrence* of thyroid cancer. But, if half of your thyroid gland still remains inside you, radioactive iodine therapy isn't all that effective because it will probably wind up causing thyroiditis (this happens about 60% of the time). Also, a radioactive iodine scan is useless because it's designed to pick up thyroid remnants that can't be seen with the naked eye. The bottom line is that the more thyroid tissue left inside you, the more potential there is for it to become cancerous, and hence, repeat all the diagnostic tests as well as surgery.

If you do wind up with a lobectomy, you may not require any thyroid hormone after surgery. The remaining lobe usually enlarges slightly and works "double time" to make enough hormone for your body.

Risks of Surgery

With an experienced surgeon who does at least one thyroidectomy a week, the risks of this surgery are minimal. At any rate, about 1% of thyroidectomy patients will experience damage to nerves leading to the voice box, which lives very close to the thyroid. There may also be some damage to the parathyroid glands, which, as discussed in chapter 1, control calcium levels. Damage can cause numbness and tingling sensations around the lips, mouth, hands, and feet. Muscle cramps and twitching, and sometimes even seizures, can occur as well. If this happens, you'll be treated with large doses of vitamin D, together with calcium supplements. Finally, as in any surgery, there is a small risk that your scar could become infected. Thyroid surgery is delicate, and it's important to have an experienced head and neck surgeon who knows what he's doing! See chapter 10 for more information.

Preparing for Surgery

As soon as the cancer is detected, your surgery date will be booked. You'll be required to check into the hospital about 12 hours prior to surgery. During this time, a hospital resident (a specialist-in-training, and in this case, a surgeon-in-training) will come to see you and walk you through the surgical procedure. He or she will take your medical history to see if you have any allergies or are on medication that may cause complications. The resident will also make sure all of your questions and concerns are answered. Hospitals are run by people, and people make mistakes. So at this point it's important that you clarify you're booked for the correct procedure and that the surgeon you were referred to is in fact the same surgeon who is operating on you.

Finally, the resident will give you a form to sign granting the hospital permission to perform surgery on you. This form is a legal document. Before you sign it, make sure you read it. Ask the resident to explain anything you don't understand on the form. If the resident can't answer one of your questions, he or she will find someone who will. Don't sign the form until all of your questions are answered. (Forms vary from state to state and country to country.)

Then, an anesthesiologist (a physician who specializes in administering anesthetic during surgery) will come to see you. He or she may ask you some of the same questions just to clarify certain information. The anesthesiologist will also walk you through the surgical procedure, instructing you to fast 12 hours prior to surgery, outlining any risks associated with the anesthetic, and telling you what to expect when going under and waking up. At this point, you should voice any concerns or ask questions. Everyone has different concerns here; there are no right or wrong questions. Again, clarify with the anesthesiologist that you are scheduled for the correct procedure with the surgeon you were referred to, and so on. Consider it double-checking.

Finally, a nurse will come in to give you an injection via intravenous to induce sleep before the actual anesthetic is given. In the morning you'll be awakened very early for your procedure and wheeled into the operating room. By this point you'll feel very groggy and see everything in a dreamlike, half-conscious state. In fact, you'll feel so drowsy, worry will be the farthest thing from your mind. Your entire neck and chest area will be painted with an antiseptic, ironically iodine. The anesthesiologist will then start the anesthetic via intravenous and tell you to count backward from 100. You won't make it to 90 before you fall into a deep sleep.

When you wake up, you'll be back in your room after having been in surgery between 2 and 5 hours. Some people feel nauseated after an anesthetic and throw up for the first few hours after they wake up. This is normal. Your neck will be completely bandaged, and you won't have any feeling in the bandaged area. This is because nerve endings are severed in the procedure. (They take several years to grow back.) You'll also find a suction tube attached to your neck which connects to a suction machine. The tube drains your neck and sucks out all of the fluid that collects after surgery (this is done with any procedure, not just a thyroidectomy!). And what about pain? Believe it or not, you're more uncomfortable from the intravenous and the suction tube than from any pain. Because your nerve endings were severed, you'll probably feel numb with a little bit of a sore throat. That's *it*—honest! You'll also be on painkillers, often over the counter, which also diminish your discomfort.

You'll be in the hospital for about four days, and then you'll be recuperating at home for one to three weeks. Plastic surgery techniques are used for closing the incision made at surgery, so the scarring is minimal and is often hidden in the natural creases of your neck. In addition, the scar is so thin that it's often easily hidden by a necklace. After about two weeks at home, your stitches will be removed and your neck may be further drained with a needle. You'll then be started on thyroid hormone permanently. An endocrinologist usually takes care of monitoring your dosage until you're bal-

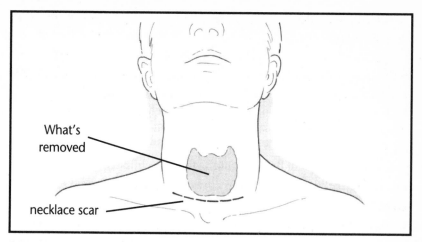

What's removed

necklace scar

Fig. 6-1 After a thyroidectomy.

Reprinted from *Nichts Gutes im Schilde Krankheiten der Schilddruse.* Copyright 1994, Georg Thieme Publishing.

anced. You may experience hypo- or hyperthyroidism until you're on the right dosage, however.

Radioactive Iodine Treatment

If you've had cancer in a secondary stage and have had a total thyroidectomy, radioactive iodine treatment is the next step after surgery. The purpose of this is for overkill—to make absolutely certain that thyroid cancer hasn't a chance of developing anywhere else in your body. Radioactive iodine destroys all thyroid cells and tissue in the body and therefore destroys all differentiated forms of thyroid cancer or normal cells that could have the potential of becoming cancerous. (Chapter 11 explains radioactive iodine in detail. If you require this treatment, make sure you read it.)

You'll be given another thyroid scan (see chapter 5) to check the success of the thyroidectomy procedure, verifying how much, if any, thyroid tissue is still left in your body. Again, you are given a "tracer" of radioactive iodine (I^{123}). Usually a slightly higher dosage is required for this test. After this follow-up scan, you will probably need a body scan, during which the imager takes pictures of your entire body to make sure the cancer hasn't spread *beyond* your thyroid.

Your doctor will take you off your thyroid replacement hormone to induce a hypothyroid state deliberately and trigger the release of thyroid stimulating hormone (TSH) into your blood. TSH will stimulate both the normal and cancerous tissue to absorb iodine, and the test becomes far more accurate. The same thing is also done when you're finally given radioactive iodine as a treatment for thyroid cancer.

Radioactive iodine treatment for thyroid cancer is a little more extreme. The typical dosage ranges between 100 and 150 millicuries. That's a lot. The reason for such a high dosage (anything over 30 millicuries) is that with thyroid cancer, the aim is to kill *all* thyroid tissue throughout your body. It's only given as a *secondary* stage of treatment, depending upon how advanced the cancer is.

After treatment, you will be kept in isolation in a private hospital room for at least two days. That means no visitors! There's almost no discomfort other than a dry mouth or tenderness in the neck. Aside from the obvious anxiety or depression you may experience from the mere thought of undergoing such an experience, you spend quiet time in the hospital reading, watching television, or talking on the telephone to family and friends.

The hospital staff brings you all your meals, towels, and so forth. You're required to urinate into a special container that fits like a "potty" over the toilet bowl. Hospital staff will then regularly enter your room and check your urine with a Geiger counter to determine the amount of radioactivity released. Once your levels of radiation are "safe" enough for you to be exposed to others, you're allowed to go home. You should probably practice the precautions outlined in chapter 11 for another couple of days until the radiation half-life is reduced considerably.

After about 10 days, you may need to undergo one more scan to make sure that the treatment has *worked*—it almost always has. Once the posttreatment test is done, you're usually home-free. Only in rare cases is treatment not successful.

It's natural to have some reservations about radioactive iodine, but it's considered a very safe and routine procedure for thyroid testing and treatment. You're in a lot more danger if you resist treatment and allow your illness to progress untreated. In fact, you probably breathe in toxins on a daily basis that are a lot more harmful. True, it is radiation to an extent, but certainly not to any dangerous degree, such as the results of exposure to radiation from the Chernobyl nuclear accident. Radioactive iodine does not cause leukemia or any other kind of cancer. Moreover, it does not cause infertility or increase your chances of having a malformed fetus, as long as you wait at least six months to get pregnant after receiving treatment.

That said, I can't tell you how many calls I've received from readers who cry on the phone because their doctors—usually primary care physicians who generally don't know a whole lot about radioactive iodine—have told them that radioactive iodine therapy can cause leukemia, breast cancer, ovarian failure, and a whole list of horrors. Any thyroid specialist will tell you *this is just not true.* I also have file folders of studies reporting the same thing. Patients who have received this therapy, including me, have been followed since the 1950s, and have not developed any more of these cancers than the general population. If your doctor tells you otherwise, he or she is just not up on the literature. Earlier studies suggested that one could expect five cases of leukemia per 1,000 patients treated with 500 millicuries of radioactive iodine—an almost unheard of amount. Essentially, saying that you're likely to develop leukemia after a standard 100 millicurie dose of radioactive iodine is as logical as saying that your chances of being hit by a car may increase after this therapy.

What *is* true, however, is that if you've had one endocrine cancer, you're statistically more at risk for other endocrine cancers such as breast cancer—but this has *nothing* to do with radioactive iodine and everything to do with genes and family history.

The only other risks being studied right now is the effect of radioactive iodine therapy on the salivary glands. There seems to be an increase in salivary gland inflammation (called sialoadenitis) following this therapy. Experts recommend sucking on lemons following the therapy to get your salivary glands working and stimulated.

In many ways, radioactive iodine is really a "miracle" cure. For more information, call the Society of Nuclear Medicine (212) 889-0717, or contact one of the thyroid foundations listed in the appendix at the back of this book.

External Radiation

If you've had a thyroidectomy and had the surrounding lymph nodes removed, in some instances your surgeon will want you to have radiotherapy, or external radiation therapy. This is the last stop on the treatment train, but it is also the most unpleasant part of your treatment. Again, the purpose of external radiation therapy is usually for overkill, a don't-even-think-of-coming-back response to thyroid cancer.

Radiation therapy may involve either cobalt beam or laser beam treatments—*not* X-ray treatments and *not* chemotherapy. (Cobalt beams are more common.) Therefore, your hair will not fall out and you will not experience any nausea or any other side effects associated with chemotherapy. Laser beams are very exact and are only directed at the area of your neck to where the cancer has spread. The concept is very simple. Laser beams give off radiation, a kind of energy that excites and kills the cells they target. If a cell is cancerous, it is also killed. The actual process, however, is a little more complex. First, you'll be referred to a radiotherapist, a doctor who specializes in radiation therapy (*not* to be confused with a radiologist, a doctor who specializes in reading X rays and diagnostic test results). The radiotherapist will then "tattoo you" by injecting a tiny dot of special dye into a precise area of your neck. The dot will look like a small, blue freckle. This dye will later be picked up by the laser beam, which will use the tattoo as an exact target for a squared-off section of your neck, predetermined by the radiotherapist. The amount of external radiation treatment is small compared with treatment for other types of cancers. A typical treatment scenario for thyroid cancer is about 30 seconds of radiation every weekday for a month. Women with breast cancer, for example, can have as much as 10 minutes of radiation every day for six months! This gives you an idea of how minimal the radiation dosage is.

After you're tattooed, you'll report a few days later to a radiation clinic, located in the hospital basement. Radiation clinics are situated in the basement because hospitals want to minimize the risk of radiation exposure to healthy people. It's really a just security measure; however, reporting to a clinic in the bowels of a hospital can feel very isolating and depressing. That's why it's important to bring someone along for support, so make sure you don't go alone.

The radiation clinic will have a number of radiotechnicians on staff who will operate the actual machinery. You'll go into a dark room and lie down on something that looks like an examination table with a device overhead. The device activates the laser beam. You'll be covered in lead blankets, and only your neck area will be exposed. The beam will then be turned on.

Although the procedure itself is painless the aftereffects are not. Knowing this in advance may not alleviate the symptoms, but it may make them more understandable and therefore more bearable.

For the first week of treatment, you probably won't feel much. By week two, the squared-off area that the beam targets will look like a very bad sunburn, and your throat will feel extremely sore. Swallowing will be very painful. As the treatment progresses, your throat will become more tender. You'll also feel quite tired by the third or fourth week of treatment, because the procedure is mentally as well as physically draining.

To relieve the symptoms, the best suggestion is to chew Aspergum continuously. This really helps. Some radiotherapists will prescribe a topical anesthetic to gargle, such as Xylocaine (pronounced ZY-loh-kane), which numbs all feeling in your throat. It tastes pretty bad, so this may not always work. To help with the sunburn symptoms, use either over-the-counter sunburn creams or ask the radiotherapist or radiotechnician on staff to recommend something. Generally, diaper-rash creams or sunburn creams that are safe for babies work quite well. Obviously, eating soft foods will be better. If you're turned off by food altogether, you could survive on a drink called Ensure, a meal supplement drink sold in drugstores or hospital pharmacies. The drink is like a sweet milkshake and tastes like the meal replacement drink from various diet programs.

As soon as the treatments are finished, you'll start to feel much better. You'll then need one more thyroid scan about three months later. After that, your treatment should be finished, and your cancer should be cured.

Dealing with the "C" Word

The most difficult part of the diagnosis is dealing with the notion of actually *having* cancer. Even though you're assured repeatedly that thyroid cancer isn't fatal and is curable almost all of the time, the stigma of cancer is still there. To make matters worse, cancer patients often find that they spend most of their time reassuring *other* people, particularly close family members and relatives. By the time they finish comforting *them* and dispelling the third-party panic that results, they have very little energy left for themselves. Pity is another problem. When others are anxious about your condition and worry about how your condition will affect *them* or fear the same predicament, their response is to pity. This emotion is characterized by an I-would-hate-for-that-to-be-me attitude. Nobody likes to be pitied. When people are supportive, however, their sympathy implies an if-that-were-me-this-is-how-I'd-like-to-be-treated attitude—a "do unto others" philosophy.

What can you do to avoid the panic and pity of others? First, find out as much information as you can about your condition before you tell *anyone* about your illness. For information and access to networks of other cancer or thyroid patients, you can call the American Cancer Society or the Canadian Cancer Society (listed in your phone directory), or contact the Thyroid Foundation of America, Inc., or the Thyroid Foundation of Canada. (See the appendix.) Hospitals usually have social workers, psychologists, or therapists who work exclusively with cancer patients. Ask your doctor to refer you to one of these professionals. It's important to talk to someone who has had experience with other cancer patients; that way your own experience won't feel so isolating, and it can be put in perspective. You can also turn to other support networks. For example, many corporations and businesses now offer a free program to their employees called the Employee Assistance Program. If you have access to this organization, you can speak to a qualified therapist in complete confidence and at your own convenience while your employer picks up the tab. These sessions are prepaid, and the program is offered as a benefit and service to employees. If your company provides the Employee Assistance Program, brochures or posters for this program are displayed on company bulletin boards with an 800 number. If you're not sure whether the program is provided, ask your human resources manager. Do take advantage of it if you can. Depending on your religious or community affiliations, there are also funded social services organizations that have social workers or therapists on hand providing assistance.

Only after you've done your own research, gathered some answers, or spoken to someone about your cancer will you be better equipped to tell people close to you about your condition.

Whom Do You Tell?

What you say is as important as who you tell. That's why it's better to break the news about your condition when you're calmer and less frightened yourself. First, you'll have to decide who you need to tell in order of priority.

It's important to tell people who are supportive. Figuring this out isn't always easy. After you've been diagnosed, make a list of who you *must* tell and a list of who you *should* tell—there's a difference. For example, if you have dependent children or a spouse, they must be told. Generally, your parents must be told (unless they're estranged or very old and the news would not do them any good). Anyone you live with or have an intimate relationship with must be told. Friends, business associates, and distant relatives should be told, but it's not imperative.

Then, list on a separate sheet of paper who you *want* to tell. This category usually includes your real friends or one best friend. Sometimes best friends are in fact family members: spouses, mothers, fathers, sisters, adult children (if you're middle-aged, for example), aunts, and cousins. Best friends are often outside the family, however. When this is the case, they're usually more objective and therefore more supportive.

It is *this* list that becomes your priority; the people you want to tell should be told before the people you must tell. You've chosen them because they're supportive and have proven themselves to you in the past. They will make you feel better, which will give you strength to tell the people who must know. Bad news is not the same as good news. You want to shout good news to the world, which means that the names on your "must," "should," and "want" lists differ drastically from the bad news lists!

When you're prepared to tackle your want list, make sure you choose your words carefully. For example, instead of saying "I have cancer," why not begin with "I have to have an operation on my thyroid gland." Then lead slowly into the reasons for the operation. That way, the information is presented in a more logical sequence rather than in an emotional sequence. Generally, the idea is to prevent someone else's panic, which will only make you feel more anxious. You can work on how to present your news by role-playing with your therapist. Or, if you have an open relationship with your doctor, you can discuss your condition and how to best present the news with him or her. After you've told the people on your want list, you could ask them to be with you when you tell the people on your must list; that way, you have support should someone take the news badly.

To handle the should list, ask someone else to tell them—someone either on your must list or want list. That way, you don't have the extra burden of speaking to people you're not that close to or don't feel like telling yourself. Sometimes, once the people close to you know about your condition, you may wish to simply disregard the should list. Usually, people on this list are told out of politeness or out of a forced sense of loyalty. Unless there's a very good reason to tell them about your diagnosis, don't. To explain absences to business associates, or coworkers, you can simply tell them you're going to the doctor for a thyroid problem and are getting some routine tests done. That's all you have to say. Otherwise, rumors and through-the-grapevine gossip may result. (Unfortunately, other people's misfortunes are always considered the best "gossip.")

What if you don't want *anyone* to know? Depending on your situation, that's okay, too (but it's a good idea to speak to a social worker at least). If you are older, without a spouse, or have grown children, you may not have to say anything. But if you're younger and are married or living with your parents, you may not have the luxury of complete privacy.

Speaking from my own experience, people who have been treated for thyroid cancer have the unusual opportunity to see all angles of the thyroid picture. Not only do they experience a variety of diagnostic procedures and treatments, but the subsequent balancing of thyroid replacement hormone can cause them to become, at times, either hyperthyroid or hypothyroid. This makes thyroid cancer patients particularly thyroid-wise, and in a sense prepares them for any future thyroid scenario. The experience also provides many patients with coping skills for health crises that may arise later on. Cancer is often what we fear most; after having dealt with it in a treatable version, we are less fearful of other potentially threatening conditions.

Women and Thyroids

Since thyroid disorders occur overall about seven times more frequently in women, thyroid disease has been labeled a "woman's disease." However, for specific diseases such as Graves', Hashimoto's, and thyroid cancer, the figure is much higher. At any rate, this labeling has presented all kinds of negative implications for women. Many doctors, thyroid organizations, and thyroid patients feel that because of this, thyroid disease was not taken seriously in the past by a predominantly male profession.

There is *some* evidence to support this belief. According to thyroid lay organizations, many family doctors across the continent are not as up-to-date on (or aware of) thyroid disease as they should be; misdiagnosis of thyroid disease, according to the perception of many thyroid patients I interviewed, is still widespread, and not a lot of information on the thyroid gland has been published for public consumption, even though one in twenty people worldwide suffer from thyroid disorders.

How has all this affected women with thyroid disorders? Until about 1980, many women were not taken seriously when they complained of thyroid symptoms to (mostly male) family doctors who were *not* up-to-date on thyroid disease. Women were told that their symptoms were phantoms, rooted in emotional psychosis. When the symptoms persisted, these women were shrugged off as "loopy" or classified as hypochondriacs. As discussed in chapter 2, many women were (and still are) referred to psychiatrists instead of endocrinologists. This general attitude in the medical community caused many women to doubt both themselves and their bodies. Worse, in the formerly male-dominated world of doctors, many women either deified their doctors or felt intimidated by them, and hence refrained from questioning diagnoses or seeking second opinions for their very real symptoms. This "good little girl" behavior generated years of unnecessary suffering for thousands of women.

It should be duly noted, however, that thyroid disease also has a reputation for being *over*diagnosed. Some doctors report that they have many patients who ascribe symptoms to their thyroid "status" that cannot be truly related to a thyroid condition. All kinds of bizarre symptoms have been blamed on the thyroid gland, when in fact these patients are found to have completely normal functioning thyroid glands.

But continuing thyroid research has yielded some interesting results for women; as many as 10% of new mothers who in the past may have been erroneously diagnosed with postpartum depression are in fact suffering from depressionlike symptoms caused by postpartum thyroiditis (discussed below and in chapter 4).

As for the noticeable lack of information available on thyroid disease, thyroid organizations now exist in the United States, Canada, Britain, and other parts of the world. Traditionally, however, thyroid disease was a terrifying experience for women who were coping with it in the dark. This fear of the disease often made the symptoms worse.

Fortunately, times are rapidly changing. As female baby boomers start families and enter middle age, they are demanding more medical research into the areas of fertility, pregnancy, and menopause. For the first time all kinds of studies are being done that measure the effects of thyroid disorders on a woman's body. Many "female problems" are now easily corrected as normal thyroid function is restored. This is good news for female thyroid patients, and future research will continue to address the unique physical concerns women have about the thyroid gland.

The purpose of this chapter is to discuss how thyroid disorders affect the female body and, in turn, how the unique female physique affects the thyroid gland.

The Menstrual Cycle

The menstrual cycle is a very special clock for women. It tells us what biological time it is, it gauges our physical and emotional states, and it alerts us to potential health problems. When any woman experiences fluctuations in her menstrual cycle, she immediately knows that something is wrong. In fact, some women can set their watches by the accuracy of their periods. This internal gauge is often an important element in detecting a thyroid problem.

The effects of thyroid hormones on menstrual periods, ovarian function, and the endocrine system in general are complex. Both hyper- and hypothyroidism can have profound effects on a woman's menstrual cycle. When you're moderately hypothyroid, your periods are heavier and longer, while cycles are often shorter. When hypothyroidism is in a more severe stage, you may experience amenorrhea, a lack of menstruation. Bleeding that requires you to change your pad or tampon every hour is considered extremely heavy, and must be followed up by a gynecological exam. This could be a sign that other causes are at work, which may be aggravating your hypothyroidism.

Consequently, there may also be problems with ovulation and conception resulting from either the hypothyroidism itself or associated hormonal changes. For example, in some women with severe hypothyroidism, their pituitary gland produces increased amounts of a hormone known as prolactin. Prolactin is normally responsible for breastmilk production. When you're not nursing, and your levels are high, your estrogen and progesterone levels are thrown off, causing your menstrual cycles to become irregular.

When you're hyperthyroid, periods are irregular (usually the cycles are longer), scanty, and shorter. Hyperthyroid women can also experience amenorrhea and generally have a difficult time getting pregnant.

Younger girls are also affected by hyper- or hypothyroidism. If they develop a thyroid condition during puberty, for example, they may have delayed menstrual function. If you have a daughter who seems to be in this situation or are in your teens yourself and have not yet experienced your period, request a thyroid function test.

By the same token, if you are currently having problems getting pregnant or are experiencing problems with your menstrual flow, it's a good idea to get your thyroid checked first before you undergo more extreme tests. Once either the hypo- or hyperthyroidism is treated, menstrual flows and fertility return to normal. For more information about menstrual cycles consult my book, *The Gynecological Sourcebook*.

Oral Contraception

This is a concern for women who are currently on oral contraceptives (OCs) and are diagnosed with a thyroid problem. First, it's important to note that if you're on OCs, you probably won't experience any change in your menstrual cycle when you're either hyper- or hypothyroid. This is because your cycle is being "run" by the oral contraceptive. However, if you've been diagnosed with either hyper- or hypothyroidism and are on thyroid hormone replacement, you can still take OCs.

To date, all studies have concluded that OCs are perfectly safe when combined with thyroid hormone replacement because they're not really a drug but an exact duplicate of a hormone your body naturally produces. In addition, doses of thyroid hormone are extremely refined, and once your medication is balanced the thyroid pills will meet your body's exact requirements. Furthermore, OCs have been refined to the point where estrogen doses are also very sensitive and very low. Although women have reported side effects when they combine their thyroid pills with Estrogen Replacement Therapy (if you have no uterus) or Hormonal Replacement Therapy (if you still have your uterus) prescribed after menopause (discussed below), OCs work nicely with thyroid hormone replacement. At any rate, if you're taking thyroid hormone replacement, you should notify your doctor, gynecologist, or whoever prescribed the OC. Conversely, if you're on OCs, you should notify your doctor, endocrinologist, or whoever prescribed thyroid hormone.

It's important to note that some side effects of combination oral contraceptives, such as weight gain, increased appetite, depression, and a long list of other vague symptoms, may be confused with a thyroid condition, or may mask one. Report any unusual symptoms to your doctor. Going off the oral contraceptive will confirm or rule out a thyroid problem in this case.

Progesterone-only contraception

There are a variety of hormonal contraceptive products that do not use estrogen, but a synthetic progesterone. Some of these products are subdermal implants (implants under the skin), such as Norplant; some are injectable, such as Depo Provera; and some are in pill form, known as the "mini-pill" or the progesterone-only oral contraceptive. While many of the side effects of these contraceptives are the same as the traditional combination oral contraceptives discussed above, one unique side effect is a highly *irregular* menstrual cycle. In this case, your irregular cycle is caused by your contraceptive and *not* your thyroid.

At any rate, regardless of whether you're on a combination hormonal contraceptive or a progesterone-only recipe, you cannot use your menstrual cycle to monitor your thyroid levels. For more information on contraception consult my book, *The Gynecological Sourcebook*, as well.

Infertility

About 30% of all female infertility is caused by hormonal factors, of which only a tiny segment is due to thyroid disorders. It's also crucial to note that you may have other factors contributing to your infertility in conjunction with a thyroid problem. If you're having difficulty conceiving, make sure your doctor rules out other causes before your problem is blamed on a thyroid condition alone. It's important to remember that infertility is always temporary when it's caused by either hyper- or hypothyroidism. As discussed above, because both hyper- and hypothyroidism interfere with the menstrual cycle, ovulation is affected as well. Generally, infertility occurs when either a hyper- or hypothyroid condition is severe and remains undiagnosed. Thyroid problems are usually caught, however, before infertility becomes a problem, and even women with severe cases of hyper- or hypothyroidism can still get pregnant. In other words, just because you're hypo- or hyperthyroid doesn't mean you won't get pregnant, so if you normally practice contraception, you should continue to do so throughout diagnosis and treatment of your thyroid problem. If, however, infertility is a side effect to your thyroid problem, it clears up as soon as you're treated and normal thyroid function resumes (presuming no other barriers to your fertility).

Another problem with hyper- or hypothyroidism which can block pregnancy is that your desire for sex can be diminished. Because of the exhaustion or fatigue that sets in, you might find that you simply don't have the energy or desire. Again, this is a temporary problem that clears up when your thyroid problem is treated.

Primary ovary failure is an autoimmune disorder—like Graves' disease and Hashimoto's thyroiditis—caused by proteins and white blood cells that attack proteins in your ovaries. This leads to a shriveling of the ovary, failure to ovulate, premature menopause, and infertility. Sometimes these autoimmune ovarian problems coexist with hypothyroidism, but this is very rare. In this case hypothyroidism might originally be suspected as the cause of infertility. However, further tests would discover primary ovary failure, a condition that exists independently of the thyroid problem.

It's important to note that hypothyroidism is more common in women with polycystic ovary syndrome, as well as women with Turner's syndrome, a genetic disorder where the ovaries do not make eggs without female hormone supplements. For more information about infertility consult my book, *The Fertility Sourcebook*.

Pregnancy

Thyroid problems during and after pregnancy are common. As discussed in chapter 3, women with a family history of thyroid disease are statistically more vulnerable to autoimmune disorders such as Graves' disease or Hashimoto's thyroiditis during their first trimester or in the first six months after delivery. Graves' disease, Hashimoto's thyroiditis, and postpartum thyroiditis are the most common thyroid conditions during or after pregnancy.

Postpartum thyroiditis is a recently discovered problem that spans the spectrum of both hyper- and hypothyroidism. This condition, which tends to occur a few months after pregnancy, may produce antibodies that damage thyroid tissue, thereby releasing thyroid hormone passively into the bloodstream and causing hyperthyroidism. Before the recovery phase, thyroid levels may fall, producing either temporary or permanent thyroid failure. Since this condition is common, occurring in 8 to 10% of all women after pregnancy, postpartum thyroid testing is usually done on all women. If you're not tested after delivery, request it. See chapter 4 for more information.

Nodules, goiters, and other thyroid-related problems can sometimes occur during pregnancy but are less common. They are discussed later in this chapter. For more information on pregnancy consult my book, *The Pregnancy Sourcebook*.

Planning Your Pregnancy

If you've been treated for hypothyroidism and are trying to get pregnant, you should get your thyroid levels checked again while you're trying to conceive. To make sure you're taking enough thyroid hormone replacement, request both a thyroid function test (free T_4 levels) as well as a TSH test. That way you minimize any possible risk to yourself or your baby from hypothyroidism during pregnancy. Since you naturally feel more tired when you're pregnant, fatigue caused by hypothyroidism could severely lower your energy levels. Again, it's important to make sure that your pregnancy symptoms aren't masking a thyroid problem, and vice versa.

If you're being treated for hyperthyroidism with radioactive iodine, you should put off trying to get pregnant for about six months. As a precaution, all doctors screen for pregnancy first before radioactive iodine is administered.

Finally, if you're taking antithyroid medications and are planning to get pregnant, you may safely become pregnant while continuing to take them, as long as you're under the supervision of a physician. This may protect the fetus from the effects of thyroid stimulating antibodies (TSA), which can cross from the mother to the baby.

How Does a Normal Thyroid Function During Pregnancy?

It's normal for a thyroid gland to enlarge slightly in pregnancy because the fetus takes iodine away from the mother. What also happens is that the mother loses more iodine in her urine while pregnant. Another reason why the gland enlarges is because human chorionic gonadotropin (hCG), a hormone formed in the placenta, can mildly stimulate the thyroid gland. Researchers have found that hCG has a very similar molecular structure to TSH (thyroid stimulating hormone). In fact, it was customary in ancient Egypt to tie a fine thread around the neck of a young bride; when it broke, it meant she was pregnant. As a precaution, however, even a modestly enlarged thyroid gland or goiter should be checked. The more iodine-deficient the mother is (especially if she lives in an iodine-deficient area), the more enlarged the thyroid becomes.

Normal, healthy, pregnant women often develop symptoms and signs that suggest hyperthyroidism, such as a rapid pulse or palpitations, sweating, and heat intolerance. This is because the metabolic rate increases in pregnancy. Despite this, hyperthyroidism only occurs in about one in a thousand pregnancies. Thyroid hormone levels also increase during pregnancy because of the high levels of estrogen a pregnant body secretes. This is due to an increase in a binding protein in the blood that holds thyroxine there. The amount of thyroxine available to the tissues, however, is *not* increased, and the increased thyroid levels would not interfere with thyroid hormone *production* in normal pregnant women.

The Baby's Thyroid

The baby's thyroid begins to function somewhere between the tenth and twelfth week of pregnancy. Thyroid hormones are important for the development of the fetal nervous system. The hormones at this stage come primarily from the baby's thyroid gland secretions; only very small amounts of the mother's thyroid hormone cross the placenta.

Iodine in the mother's diet also crosses the placenta and is used by the fetal thyroid gland to make thyroid hormone. Iodine deficiency can cause newborn hypothyroidism or mental retardation and is a major health problem in underdeveloped countries. But since there is an overabundance of iodine in the North American diet, disorders caused by a lack of dietary iodine don't happen here. Fetal thyroid disease is discussed in chapter 9.

Thyroid Disease During Pregnancy

If you are hypothyroid or are taking thyroid hormone replacement from a thyroid condition prior to pregnancy, the thyroid hormone thyroxine—the usual treatment—is fine. Very little thyroxine crosses from the mother to the fetus. Sometimes a change in dosage is needed because requirements for thyroxine can increase during pregnancy; it's normal to require as high as a 40 to 50% increase in your dosage. In this case doctors generally monitor the TSH level anyway and will increase your dose as necessary.

If hypothyroidism is suspected *while* you're pregnant, your doctor will give you a TSH test. Just as in nonpregnant women, your

TSH levels will be increased if you're hypothyroid, and you'll be treated with thyroxine. Sometimes pregnancy itself can mask hypothyroid symptoms. For example, constipation, puffiness, and fatigue are all traits of pregnancy. If you develop these traits, your hypothyroidism is probably not that severe, but the symptoms will persist after delivery.

Hyperthyroidism during pregnancy is more complex, and when it does happen it's usually due to Graves' disease. Diagnosis and treatment of hyperthyroidism during pregnancy presents some unique fetal and maternal considerations, however. The risk of miscarriage and stillbirth is increased if hyperthyroidism goes untreated. A 1995 study showed that women with antithyroid antibodies had a 32% risk of miscarriage compared to a 16% risk in women without this antibody. Miscarriage risk also goes up as you age. Furthermore, the overall risks to the mother and baby increase if the disease persists or is first recognized late in pregnancy.

As in nonpregnant women, specific hyperthyroid symptoms usually indicate a problem, but again, some of the classic symptoms such as heat intolerance or palpitations can mirror classic pregnancy traits. Symptoms such as bulgy eyes or a pronounced goiter indicate Graves' disease. But because radioactive iodine scans or treatment are *never* performed in pregnancy, hyperthyroidism can only be confirmed through a blood test in this case.

Radioactive iodine scans are sometimes accidentally performed on pregnant women. This can happen if you don't know you're pregnant: for example, women on oral contraceptives can get pregnant, or early pregnancy tests can turn out negative, even though the patient is really positive. But when you're in obvious stages of pregnancy or know for certain that you're pregnant, no competent, licensed doctor would suggest a radioactive iodine scan. However, if by some chance a thyroid scan is done while you are in the early stages of pregnancy (during the first trimester), the amount of radioactive iodine given in a *scan* alone will not harm the fetus. In fact, the amount of radioactivity here that would enter the fetus is just barely above the normal amount of radioactivity present in the air we normally breathe.

On the other hand, if radioactive iodine *treatment* is accidentally given during early pregnancy, the amount of radiation could be enough to damage the fetus. In this case, you should seek counseling and may want to consider a therapeutic abortion, which is legal. (It should be noted, though, that completely normal infants *have* been born under these circumstances.)

If by some fluke radioactive iodine treatment is accidentally given after the first trimester, the baby's thyroid gland may be destroyed, but this is treatable at birth with thyroid hormone replacement. In this situation you wouldn't have to terminate the pregnancy. Accidents like this happen in extremely unusual, even bizarre circumstances. Sometimes lab mix-ups happen and test tubes are confused. This kind of mix-up could coincide with a woman who carries small, has no pregnancy symptoms, and simply doesn't notice she's pregnant.

Otherwise, for all other cases of hyperthyroidism in pregnancy, the treatment is antithyroid medication. Propylthiouracil or methimazole is most commonly used, but propylthiouracil is the one usually used during pregnancy because it does not cross the placenta as easily as methimazole. The antithyroid medication in pregnancy is first used to control the hyperthyroidism. Afterward, the aim is to administer the lowest dose possible to maintain the thyroid hormone levels in the high-normal, or maximum-without-risk, range. This way, smaller doses of medication pose minimum risk to the baby. Another reason why antithyroid drugs are given in low doses is because your immune system is so depressed in pregnancy that the low dose doesn't affect the baby's thyroid as it might when a high dose is given. With higher doses, the drugs cross the placenta into the baby's bloodstream and can ultimately affect the baby's thyroid. Since TSAs also cross the placenta, they can cause fetal hyperthyroidism, which is very dangerous and may even cause fetal death. Therefore, the propylthiouracil, by suppressing the fetal thyroid, actually benefits the fetus.

Sometimes women find they're allergic to propylthiouracil. If this happens, methimazole is used instead. When there's a problem with both drugs, a thyroidectomy during the second trimester may be done; this is rare, though. In general, surgery is avoided during pregnancy because it can trigger a miscarriage.

Hyperthyroidism often becomes milder as the pregnancy progresses. When this happens, antithyroid medication can be tapered off slowly as the pregnancy reaches full term, and often normal thyroid function resumes after delivery.

When Graves' disease is the cause of hyperthyroidism in pregnancy, the hyperthyroidism will need to be controlled throughout pregnancy to avoid either severe hyperthyroidism or complications during labor and delivery. Beta blockers (heart medication) such as propanalol are added to propylthiouracil, which can be continued safely during breastfeeding.

Finding a Solitary Thyroid Nodule in Pregnancy

If you discover a lump on your thyroid gland in pregnancy, investigation and treatment vary depending on what stage you're at in your pregnancy. If you're in the first trimester, a needle biopsy will be done to determine whether the lump is benign or malignant. A malignancy means that surgery would probably be performed during the second trimester, which is considered the safest time for surgery. If a cancerous nodule is confirmed in the second trimester, surgery may still be performed if there's time. Otherwise, you might simply have to wait until you deliver. As discussed in chapter 6, thyroid cancer grows very slowly, and the extra few months won't make a difference in the overall treatment scenario.

If, however, a nodule is first discovered in the second or third trimester, investigation and treatment can probably wait until you deliver. Then you'd be able to have a scan.

Postpartum Thyroid Disease

As discussed in chapter 4, after delivery, you can be caught off guard by an autoimmune disease such as Graves' disease or Hashimoto's thyroiditis, particularly if you have a family history of thyroid disease. In these cases you would undergo normal treatment for either disease. If you developed Graves' disease after delivery, however, you would not have to discontinue breast-feeding, since propylthiouracil doesn't cross into your milk. If you had developed Graves' disease during pregnancy, the condition can get worse after delivery unless antithyroid drugs are continued.

If you were diagnosed and successfully treated for Graves' disease prior to your pregnancy, sometimes you can suffer a relapse after delivery. But depending on the severity of Graves' disease after delivery, some women can opt to postpone treatment until they're finished breast-feeding.

Postpartum thyroiditis, which occurs in 5 to 18% of all postpartum women, lasting 6 to 9 months, is often the culprit behind postpartum depression or the maternal blues. However, it should be noted that during the first three months after delivery, maternal blues symptoms such as fatigue, depression, memory loss, and weak concentration are common and often have nothing to do with a woman's thyroid hormone levels. In addition, not every woman who has an emotional disorder after pregnancy necessarily has a thyroid problem. Recently, a clinical study was done on a group of women who had postpartum psychoses (a severe, but uncommon postpartum psychiatric condition). None of the women in the study was found to have any kind of thyroid problem. Nevertheless, if you or someone you know is experiencing emotional difficulties after delivery, it's perfectly reasonable to request a thyroid test, just in case.

The Breast Connection

At one time (after the first edition of this book was published), there were some confusing reports as to whether thyroid disease was associated with breast cancer. *It's not.* If you have a strong family history of endocrine cancers, which includes thyroid cancer (although a large percentage of thyroid cancer is caused by an external trigger, such as X-ray therapy in childhood or radioactive iodine fallout), then, statistically, you're more at risk for developing an endocrine cancer of *some kind*. Thyroid hormone replacement pills do not cause breast cancer, nor does radioactive iodine therapy cause breast cancer, which is based on 50 years of tracking patients who received it. While, for the most part, there are relatively few absolutes about the causes of breast cancer, right now, thyroid sufferers do not appear to have a higher incidence of breast cancer than women in the general population.

There are certain breast functions and breast conditions that are affected by thyroid diseases and treatments. If you're breast-feeding, you shouldn't undergo a radioactive iodine scan (thyroid scan) or be treated with radioactive iodine. Radioactive isotopes are secreted into the breast milk and can be passed on to your child.

The antithyroid drug propylthiouracil, *can* be used when you're breast-feeding, for the same reasons discussed earlier. Thyroxine is also safe. Although it's also secreted into the milk, as long as your dosage is balanced it won't harm your child in any way.

Some of you may have been diagnosed with fibrocystic breast condition. Essentially, this is an umbrella term that refers to six separate benign breast conditions that have absolutely nothing to do with each other. At any rate, one of these conditions is known as *non-cyclical breast pain*. This is *anatomical* (something inside the breast *itself* is causing the pain) rather than hormonal, so it does not necessarily disappear with menopause or your period, the way *hormonal* breast pain would. Often, this pain is caused by a large cyst. In fact, many women are simply prone to painful cysts. Because of this, women have come to believe that fibrocystic breast condition equals painful, lumpy breasts. *This is not true at all.* But women with this particular breast problem, who are told they have fibrocystic breast condition, may be put on an iodine treatment, which has proven helpful. This therapy appears to be more widely used outside the United States. Many U.S. breast specialists are not aware of iodine therapy for *any* breast condition whatsoever.

Interestingly, studies now show that the ovaries and *breasts* also need iodine—just like the thyroid gland. (One researcher has called the breast a "big thyroid gland.") Women with painful cysts in their breasts *have* shown tremendous improvement with this kind of iodine treatment. The catch is, if you have iodine treatment for breast pain caused by cysts, your *thyroid gland* can become overactive. Or, if you're on thyroid medication already, the iodine can interfere with it. Just make sure your thyroid condition and breast condition are managed by the same doctor. If you're on this iodine treatment, you should have your thyroid hormone levels tested every six months, and your doctor should feel your neck area to rule out signs of a goiter.

Menopause

Menopause is a Greek term taken from the words *menos* which means "month," and *pause* which means "arrest"—the arrest of the menstrual cycle. Natural menopause and *menarche* (the first menstrual period) have a lot in common: they are both *gradual* processes that women ease into. A woman doesn't suddenly wake up to find herself in menopause any more than a young girl wakes up to find herself in puberty. However, when menopause occurs *surgically* as the by-product of an *oophorectomy* (surgical removal of the ovaries), or ovarian failure occurs (resulting from cancer therapy or a hysterectomy, for example), it can be an extremely jarring process. These women may indeed wake up one morning to find themselves in menopause, and as a result, will suffer far more noticeable and severe menopausal symptoms than their natural menopause counterparts. It is because of *surgical* menopause that *Hormonal Replacement Therapy* (HRT) and *Estrogen Replacement Therapy* (ERT or "unopposed estrogen") have become such hotly debated issues in women's health. The loss of estrogen, in particular, leads to drastic changes in the body's chemistry that trigger a more aggressive aging process. Replacing these hormones will offset the aging process, which is an appropriate therapy for millions of women who are in surgical menopause, and who should not be "aging before their time."

When menopause occurs naturally, it tends to take place anywhere between the ages of 48 and 52, but it can occur as early as your late 30s, or as late as your mid-50s. When menopause occurs *before* 35, it is technically considered "early menopause." In any event, the average age of menopause is 50 to 51.

Socially, the word "menopause" refers to a process, not a precise moment in the life of your menstrual cycle. But medically, the word "menopause" does *indeed* refer to one precise moment: the date of your last period. However, the events preceding and following menopause amount to a huge change for women both physically and socially.

As you approach menopause, a hormone called follicle stimulating hormone (FSH) peaks. FSH is responsible for kickstarting your menstrual cycle and reminding your ovaries to make estrogen. However, since your ovaries are closing down for business, estrogen levels will keep dropping, while FSH levels will keep rising. This drop in estrogen and peak in FSH is what causes the range of menopausal symptoms that include skin dryness (particularly vaginal dryness), hot flashes, mood swings, depression, and a long list of other unpleasant symptoms. Unfortunately, many of the symptoms of menopause mimic the symptoms of either hyper- or hypothyroidism. This can create a menopausal misdiagnosis of nightmarish proportions.

FSH and estrogen work the same way that TSH and thyroxine do. FSH, like TSH, is released from the pituitary gland. In the same way that thyroid hormone inhibits TSH, the female hormone, estrogen, inhibits FSH. And, just as synthetic thyroid hormone is the answer to high TSH levels in someone who is hypothyroid, small amounts of synthetic estrogen are given to women to alleviate menopausal symptoms caused by the rise in FSH. When estrogen levels are balanced, FSH levels drop, which is the concept behind the Pill.

When women enter menopause and begin to experience menopausal symptoms, they are usually given Premarin, the most commonly used synthetic estrogen product. Premarin is fine for a woman with a normal thyroid gland, but in women on thyroxine or those who have a personal or family history of thyroid disease, it's important to request a thyroid function test at least once during menopause. Because hyper- or hypothyroid symptoms can be mistaken for menopausal symptoms, you don't want to end up with too high an estrogen dose when what you really need is thyroid hormone replacement. So far, studies of age-specific incidence of thyroid disease do *not* show a rise of hyperthyroidism in menopausal years. However, as baby boomers enter menopause, these statistics may change.

Osteoporosis

One of the most common questions women on thyroid hormone ask is: What's the link between thyroid disease and osteoporosis? Contrary to what most women think, the link has *nothing* to do with calcitonin, which the thyroid also produces, discussed in chapter 1. So ladies, here's the real story to set the record straight.

Thyroid hormone is something our body uses literally from head to toe. In general, anyone with too much thyroid hormone in their system is vulnerable to bone loss. That's because thyroid hormone will "speed up" or "slow down" bone cells just as it will speed or slow other parts of our bodies, such as our metabolism. Osteoblasts are the cells responsible for building bone, while osteoclasts are cells that remove old bone so the new bone can be replaced. When you're hyperthyroid, osteoclasts get overstimulated; in short, they go nuts. They begin to remove bone faster than it can be replaced by the osteoblasts, which are not affected by hyperthyroidism. So you wind up with too much bone removed which results in bone loss.

However, once your hyperthyroidism is treated, and your thyroid hormone replacement medication is balanced, the risk is gone. But, as we all know, finding the right dosage can be tricky, especially since our thyroid hormone dosage requirements change as we age, gain or lose weight, and so on. What experts recommend is to make sure you have your thyroid hormone levels checked every year so you can adjust your dosage accordingly. Women who have had a thyroidectomy to treat thyroid cancer need to be on a slightly higher dosage of thyroid hormone to suppress all TSH activity, which means that dosage balancing can be especially challenging. What I recommend in all cases (particularly in this one), is to *insist* that your doctor prescribes a thyroid hormone tablet with *precise dosing*—as most of the brand name tablets offer, such as Synthroid, Levoxyl, Levothroid, or Eltroxin (in Canada only). Some women may do better on 137 micrograms instead of 125 or 150, for example.

Thyroid, Osteoporosis, and Menopause

The thyroid-osteoporosis issue becomes exacerbated for postmenopausal women, particularly those who have gone through menopause only in the last seven years. As you may already know, estrogen, which is made by the ovaries, is responsible for helping our bodies absorb calcium needed to maintain bone mass. When our calcium levels are low, our bodies get it from our bones, which contributes to further bone loss. When you're hyperthyroid and in menopause, it's a combo platter that's very hard on the bones.

How Can I Prevent Osteoporosis When I Have a Thyroid Problem?

First, get that thyroid problem or thyroid dosage under control as quickly as possible. Second, if you have no history of breast cancer, consider going on Hormone Replacement Therapy (HRT). HRT not only halts bone loss, but protects you from heart disease, which claims more women's lives than any other illness. Third, eat well and exercise. Calcium *can* be eaten; exercise will build bone mass! See chapter 13 for details on nutrition, which includes the appropriate amount of calcium for women at all stages of their lives.

What If I Cannot Be On HRT?

If you cannot be on HRT because of your medical history, diet and exercise can really do wonders. In rare cases, calcitonin injections can be given to boost calcium levels. Right now, sodium etidronate, a substance used in many parts of the world, including the U.K., can also prevent bone loss but it is still considered experimental in North America.

Beyond 60

If you've been diagnosed with a thyroid disorder before or during menopause and are on thyroid hormone replacement, it's a good idea to have your thyroid tested regularly. Dosage requirements change as you age, and too high a dosage can cause symptoms of hyperthyroidism and place an unnecessary burden on the heart.

However, it's also very common for women to develop a thyroid disorder after 60, particularly hypothyroidism. In fact, approximately 20% of the over-60 population is clinically hypothyroid, and women in this age group are about four times as likely to develop hypothyroidism than men. One reason is because immune system abnormalities are much more common in women than men, and as the immune system ages, its function declines. Another more obvious reason is because women statistically live longer than men, which increases the women-to-men ratio. Unfortunately, diagnosing any thyroid disorder after 60 can be difficult because the symptoms of both hypo- and hyperthyroidism can be misinterpreted.

For example, hypothyroid symptoms such as an intolerance to cold, weight gain, constipation, and apathetic behavior are also mimic symptoms of aging. Similarly, hyperthyroid symptoms such as palpitations, nervousness, sweating, weight loss, and muscle weakness are also seen as aging symptoms. If you're experiencing some of these symptoms, it's always a good idea to request a thyroid function test. Hypothyroidism or hyperthyroidism would confirm either a decrease or increase in thyroid hormone.

Treating hypothyroidism after 60 is relatively simple; you're put on thyroid hormone replacement. However, your dosage may be lower than a younger patient's for the reasons mentioned above. In milder cases of hypothyroidism, you may not need immediate treatment unless you're experiencing definite symptoms. Hashimoto's disease is usually a common cause of hypothyroidism after 60.

Hyperthyroidism after age 60 can have one of four causes: Graves' disease, a multinodular goiter, subacute thyroiditis (see chapter 4), or a solitary toxic adenoma (see chapter 5). Occasionally, Hashimoto's disease can cause hyperthyroid symptoms as well. Treatment is then the same as it is for all hyperthyroid patients, but antithyroid drugs are used more often after age 60 than before age 60.

The Hiroshima Maiden Syndrome

Hiroshima Maiden Syndrome is a term head and neck surgeons use when referring to North American women who have been burned as a result of electrolysis treatments to the face and neck. Electrolysis is considered to be a safe and effective way to remove unwanted hair from these areas, but about 10 years ago head and neck surgeons began to see a significant number of women who were badly scarred and burned by either sloppy or excessive electrolysis treatments. Ironically, these burns mimicked those seen on victims of the atomic bomb in Hiroshima. Hence, the term *Hiroshima Maiden Syndrome* was born, since only females are involved with electrolysis. What does this have to do with the thyroid gland?

Some surgeons report treating "Hiroshima Maidens" for nodules on the thyroid gland; in some cases the nodules prove to be malignant. This is similar to the X-ray therapy scenario described in chapter 5.

Whatever the reason, if you are currently having electrolysis treatments to your face or neck areas, or are considering it, here are some precautions to follow:

1. Make sure you check out alternative methods of hair removal, such as waxing, tweezing, or bleaching.
2. If you still feel electrolysis is the best solution for you, make sure you go to a reputable salon with a licensed technician. Before you undergo treatment, ask for references and request a visit to past customers.
3. Try to go to a salon recommended to you by a close friend or relative.
4. If you're having trouble finding a good salon, seek out a derma-

tologist (a doctor who specializes in skin problems) and see if he or she has some suggestions or can recommend a reputable salon where you can have electrolysis done.

Every age carries special considerations for female thyroid patients. Awareness of some of these issues and healthy discussions with your family doctor, gynecologist, or endocrinologist can prevent thyroid disorders or complications to diagnosis and treatment of thyroid disorders. Most women see at least two doctors simultaneously. Chapter 10 discusses how you can make your various doctor visits more effective and hence prevent possible misdiagnoses or simple misunderstandings related to thyroid problems.

The next chapter will briefly discuss the unique concerns of men. Obviously, there are a number of complicated concerns for women with thyroid disorders; the male issues are not nearly as numerous or complex. But if you are a man with a thyroid disorder, accurate information is important for you, too.

Thyroid Disorders and Men

Although the symptoms of thyroid disorders are the same in men and women in general, there are some unique physical and emotional obstacles men can experience when they are diagnosed. The purpose of this chapter is to outline how thyroid disorders can affect both the male physique and the male psyche. This chapter also documents the experience of one man's struggle with Hashimoto's disease. While Hashimoto's disease is a relatively uncommon thyroid problem in men, this particular man is quite average in age and occupation. By highlighting his unique thyroid experience, we can gain greater insight into the universal problems men with thyroid disease experience.

But It's Not a Manly Disease!

When it comes to thyroid problems, women outperform men about five to one. As we discussed in chapter 7, it is because of this statistic that thyroid disease has been branded a "woman's disease." This doesn't mean that men do not develop thyroid problems. Out of roughly 13 million North Americans with thyroid disorders, 20% are men. Despite this, the most common emotion men can experience when they're diagnosed is embarrassment. "I thought *women* were the only ones that got this!" and "My *father* never had this problem!" might be a man's typical response.

Another layer to the embarrassment has to do with the fact that thyroid disorders involve hormones. Typically, the word *hormone* is not something men feel comfortable with; hormones are a woman's domain. Although the thyroid certainly has nothing to do with sexual hormones, men are nevertheless intimidated by the prospect of hormonal therapy of *any* kind.

This male embarrassment over thyroid disease was blatant with the media's response to former president George Bush's bout with Graves' disease. Although both the president and Mrs. Bush were diagnosed with Graves' disease and both received radioactive iodine treatment, much of the news coverage surrounded only *Mrs.* Bush's treatment and diagnosis; the president's thyroid illness seemed to generate less press and was swept under the carpet by the White House staff. Even the statistically minuscule coincidence of both the president and first lady having Graves' disease was hushed up. This is odd, considering that former president Ronald Reagan made headlines when he had a polyp removed from his bowels. In fact, the entire world was treated to play-by-play coverage of the minor surgery President Reagan underwent to get his polyp removed. Isn't a bowel polyp more compromising and embarrassing than Graves' disease? And isn't radioactive iodine treatment more newsworthy than minor surgery? Apparently not. It's likely that the White House did not want to expose the president's stress levels, since Graves' disease is an autoimmune disorder that is often triggered by stress. Indeed, what position is more stressful than that of the presidency? But it's also possible that in the eyes of the White House staff, it was thought that President Bush was better served by downplaying his thyroid illness; they didn't want him to appear weak by falling prey to the same illness as his wife. In fact, George Bush's illness may have contributed to his obvious exhaustion in the final days of the 1992 presidential campaign and to his sluggish and rather delayed entry into the race, a complaint of many Bush/Quayle campaign officials. Since dosages of thyroid hormone replacement sometimes need to be adjusted in the first couple of years after treatment—all part of the thyroid medication balancing act—and given the stressful nature of Bush's lifestyle, it's entirely possible that George Bush required frequent dosage adjustment. He may have suffered bouts of hypothyroidism from too low a thyroxine dosage, which in turn would have caused sluggishness and low energy levels. Or, he may have had further rounds of hyperthyroidism from too high a thyroxine dosage, causing exhaustion.

At any rate, we'll never know how much of an impact Graves' disease had on President Bush and the collapse of the Republican reign. Am I implying that if Bush had not suffered from Graves' disease and had begun campaigning early with the same physical stamina as Clinton had, he would have managed to win a second term? Certainly not! The point is, President Bush's illness has put thyroid disease on the map, transforming it from a "woman's disease" to one that is "presidential."

The Isolation Factor

After the possible embarrassment of thyroid disease wears off, men face another very real problem of isolation. When a woman has a thyroid problem, it's not difficult for her to find a thyroid confidante. Many people either know of or are related to a woman with a thyroid disorder. For a man, it's difficult to find a comrade who's in the same thyroid boat.

The best place to turn in these circumstances is to thyroid organizations. Either the Thyroid Foundation of America, Inc., or the Thyroid Foundation of Canada provides regular public education lectures and offers a networking service where thyroid patients can meet one another. Unfortunately, most of the men involved in these organizations are often supporting their wives, relatives, or female friends; however, they can still make powerful allies for male thyroid patients seeking support. Yet the main purpose, of course, is to find out more information on thyroid disorders and seek comfort in knowing that you're not the only man to experience this. It should also be noted, however, that men generally do not like to admit to being ill at all. Delayed thyroid diagnosis in men is often due simply to an unwillingness, on their part, to see a doctor.

What Kind of Thyroid Problems are Men Prone to?

According to some statistics, it's reported that 50% of the men who develop thyroid nodules have thyroid cancer. (See chapters 5 and 6.) Some of the diagnoses are a result of previous exposure to X-ray therapy, discussed in chapter 5. But usually, the reasons why thyroid cancer develops in men is idiopathic, or unknown. The remaining proportion of male thyroid patients suffer from a hodgepodge of thyroid diseases ranging from Graves' disease to Hashimoto's thyroiditis. Men who come from a family with a history of thyroid disease are more prone statistically to develop thyroid disorders than men who have no family history of thyroid disease. However, as described in the scenario later in this chapter, it's not unheard of for men with a clean thyroid family history to develop thyroid disease.

Stress is also a major factor in triggering some autoimmune thyroid diseases such as Graves' disease and Hashimoto's disease. Men often feel stress far more than women for a number of reasons. First, their roles and expectations in the business and professional world are often more demanding because men feel the pressures of having to be the breadwinner. Men who leave the office on time or request parental leave are often looked down on by their employers. As a result, long hours away from home and the fear of being unsuccessful can create tremendous stress for men. In addition, men still are not encouraged to express their feelings in the same way that women do. As a result, pent-up frustrations and anger can lie dormant in a man's emotional psyche for a very long time and make his stress worse. These kinds of stresses make men far more serious candidates for heart attacks and strokes, however, and thyroid problems are sometimes missed when routine tests are run during physical exams. If you come from a family with a history of thyroid problems, it's generally a good idea to request a thyroid function test every five years. You should also self-examine your neck and throat area every year for unusual lumps (nodules) that protrude, since thyroid cancer is prevalent among male thyroid patients.

However, if you don't have a history of thyroid disease in your family, it's not likely that you would develop a thyroid problem (but there is a possibility). A thyroid function test in this case wouldn't be necessary unless you experience specific symptoms of either hypo- or hyperthyroidism. Be aware that symptoms for men can include sexual dysfunction, described below.

Hyperthyroidism and Male Reproduction

Since thyroid hormone affects several tissues, too much thyroid hormone can have a profound effect on the male reproductive system. Men with hyperthyroidism may complain of impotence or find that their breasts are enlarging, a condition known as gynecomastia. Some men may also experience low sperm count and thus sterility. If a young adolescent male develops hyperthyroidism, he may experience a delay in development during normal puberty; facial and pubic hair may not develop, nor would his genitals enlarge. (If you have a son who's not developing normally at puberty, it's a good idea to get his thyroid checked. Once the hyperthyroidism is treated however, normal development should resume.)

There has been controversy in the medical community over whether hyperthyroidism influences male reproductive functions. Some doctors feel that any interruption in male reproductive functioning is extremely rare. However, a recent study on testicular function in men between 18 and 45 years of age yielded some astonishing results.

Out of nine men with hyperthyroidism and goiters caused by Graves' disease, six of them complained of poor erections or impotence occurring after their hyperthyroid symptoms manifested. The sperm count of these same men was then measured against the sperm counts of males the same age with normal thyroid function. The sperm counts of the hyperthyroid men were significantly lower, and it was concluded that an excess of thyroid hormone adversely affected sperm production in these hyperthyroid men. The study also found that testosterone (the male sex hormone) and luteinizing hormone, or LH (the male pituitary hormone), were significantly reduced in these same six men. It was the reduced levels of testosterone in these men that caused low sperm count and impotence. Yet low testosterone levels can also cause breast enlargement, experienced by some men with thyroid disorders. This means, of course, that statistically six out of nine hyperthyroid males may experience sterility.

If you do suffer from impotence or low sperm count, get your thyroid tested, just in case. If it turns out that you do have a thyroid problem, the treatment is simple and your sexual potency should be restored with normal thyroid function.

"Before I Was Diagnosed, I Lived My Whole Life Without Knowing What a Thyroid Was!"

These are the words of John, a 45-year-old recently retired IBM systems engineer who was diagnosed with Hashimoto's disease three years ago. Prior to his diagnosis he was earning roughly six figures per year, working long hours on multimillion dollar accounts in a very stressful environment. He was also beginning a new relationship with a woman he would later marry. "I was a typical baby boomer," he says.

John first began to notice symptoms of thyroid disease when he was 40 years old. He experienced odd physical and emotional symptoms he simply attributed to job burnout. He had chronic indigestion and constipation, shortness of breath, chest pain, and heart palpitations. He also suffered from anxiety attacks. These attacks were so extreme that he would wake up in the middle of the night feeling as though he would explode. At times he would pound against a piece of furniture simply to release the unexplainable tension. To aggravate matters further, John felt unusually tired, lethargic, and depressed. "I had feelings of gloom and doom. I seemed to lack the ability to care about anything or anyone," he reflects.

The symptoms started to affect John's work. "A man in my position," he says, "was expected to give 100% at all times—98% wasn't good enough." Confused about his symptoms, John decided to tackle his condition as though it were a systems engineering problem. He documented all of his health problems on paper, no matter how trivial they seemed, and then made an appointment with his family doctor. When he met with his doctor, John handed him his list of symptoms. The doctor was alarmed by the symptoms that John attributed to excessive stress, and instructed John to take an immediate two-week leave of absence from his job.

John followed his doctor's advice and did take time off, but his symptoms didn't improve. After two weeks he returned to work, where he felt he was being perceived by his coworkers as weak—someone who was cracking under pressure, someone who couldn't take the heat. John decided to see a psychiatrist, and after several sessions, he was convinced that his symptoms were purely stress-related and decided to take an early retirement package from IBM.

After resting and reading for several weeks, John's symptoms only got worse. He couldn't get enough sleep, even though he was sleeping 15 hours a night. Despite his active lifestyle, John gained about 20 pounds, and his friends commented that his face looked puffy. His eyes became bulgy as well, but he had suffered in the past from a variety of eye problems and poor eyesight, so he thought nothing of it. Finally, after a few months of retirement, John returned to his family doctor and insisted on a thorough blood test *before* another exam. It was at this point that John's T$_3$, T$_4$, and TSH levels were checked. The test showed that John's T$_3$ and T$_4$ levels were extremely low and that his TSH levels were high, a classic sign of hypothyroidism. However, the doctor merely stated that he suspected a thyroid problem.

The doctor told John that, given his symptoms, he would have routinely screened John for a thyroid disorder, but since John was male, the doctor had felt a thyroid condition was highly unlikely. He further explained that it was quite unusual for a man to have this problem. John was immediately referred to an endocrinologist, who repeated a thyroid level blood test and had him undergo both a thyroid imaging test and a radioactive iodine uptake test. The endocrinologist also found that John had quite a prominent goiter. Within 13 days John was diagnosed with chronic lymphocytic thyroiditis—Hashimoto's disease—and was prescribed 0.15 milligrams of thyroid hormone replacement. His symptoms began to disappear in a few days. John was told that his Hashimoto's disease was quite severe. As discussed in chapter 3, a severe case of hypothyroidism can lead to serious heart problems (remember John's chest pains and palpitations).

Ironically, nobody in John's family had a history of thyroid disease, and although he was well read and well educated, John had never even heard of the thyroid gland prior to his diagnosis. Hence, he didn't know that thyroid disease was reputed to be a woman's disease. "Instead," he recalls, "I felt pissed off that my doctor would rule out a thyroid test just because I was a man. His delay in testing my thyroid gland caused me a lot of unnecessary suffering." Yet because John felt so relieved to discover that his symptoms were linked to a *physical* condition and that he could be cured, embarrassment over his condition was not a factor.

Today, John says he feels better than he ever has before. After his diagnosis he also sought out a thyroid organization but has yet to meet another man with a thyroid problem.

What can we learn from John's experience? For one thing, there are still some biased attitudes about men and thyroid disorders that need to be exorcised from within the medical community. Although thyroid function tests are generally performed widely in both men and women, John's story clearly indicates that this isn't *always* the case. As John's own doctor said, had John been a woman, the doctor would have connected the symptoms to a thyroid problem much more quickly. Also more research needs to be done into the effects of thyroid hormone on the male physique. If research can pinpoint more definite "male" symptoms, misdiagnosis of thyroid disorders in men could be prevented.

However, thyroid disorders in infancy or childhood do not favor either sex and seem to occur with roughly the same frequency for both female and male children. Thyroid problems in children are discussed in the next chapter.

When It's Your Child

Although thyroid disease occurs less frequently in children and teenagers than in adults, it is still considered a common cause of disease in these age groups. When your child's thyroid is not working properly, the effects differ from those seen in an adult; hyper- or hypothyroidism can interfere with growth and development, for example. Children who come from families with a history of thyroid disease are more prone to developing thyroid disorders than children born to families with no such history. Therefore, it's important to alert your family doctor or pediatrician to any kind of thyroid history; that way, the doctor can look out for changes in your child's growth patterns and perhaps nip any thyroid problem in the bud before it manifests into more severe symptoms.

Sometimes thyroid trouble is more difficult to recognize in a child than in an adult; many children are less likely to complain or ask for help when they feel sick. Nor do they understand the difference between normal and abnormal symptoms. It's usually up to someone else to recognize the problem for them. Things to look for are an increase in irritability or hyperactivity, particularly during mealtimes or bedtime. (This sort of hyperactivity should not be confused with a child who has been diagnosed as hyperactive, a common childhood behaviorial disorder.) Teachers often notice attitude changes in school, such as poor concentration, shaky hands, and poor handwriting. If there's a change in growth rate, point out your concerns to a pediatrician, who will determine whether the change is normal or abnormal.

Some children are extremely vocal and will let you know when they're sick. In this case, ask the child to carefully relay all of his or her symptoms to you, no matter how trivial the symptoms seem. Then, if you suspect a thyroid problem, you can alert your doctor as soon as possible. (At the end of this chapter I've provided some sample questions to ask your child if you suspect thyroid disease.)

Thyroid disease can also occur at birth or in the womb, although this is rare. When this is the case, your doctor will alert you to the problem, and treatment usually corrects the problem. The purpose of this chapter is to explain the type of thyroid disorders that can occur in infants and children, as well as outline some of the treatment options available.

Fetal Thyroid Disease

Hypothyroidism

Antithyroid medications, iodine, and sometimes maternal thyroid antibodies can cross the placenta and cause hypothyroidism in the baby. Plain iodine, which is present in medications such as cough syrup can cause a goiter in the fetus, making delivery difficult or causing respiratory obstruction. For this reason, iodine-containing drugs should never be used in pregnancy except in the case of extreme hyperthyroidism, which is sometimes called thyroid storm.

Unfortunately, there is no simple blood test to assess the baby's thyroid function in the womb, although measurements of thyroid hormone or TSH levels in the amniotic fluid sac have been used in research studies. Plain X rays can show delayed bone development in fetal hypothyroidism, but this test is usually not recommended because the X ray itself can cause more damage to the fetus than the underlying condition. Screening for hypothyroidism at birth, now done routinely in North America on *all* newborns, is still the best method for determining whether your baby is hypothyroid and whether the infant needs short-term or long-term treatment in the form of thyroid hormone replacement.

Hyperthyroidism

When a fetus is hyperthyroid, the condition is known as fetal thyrotoxicosis. This happens when maternal thyroid-stimulating antibodies cross the placenta, as in the case of Graves' disease. Fetal hyperthyroidism is unusual, though. In most cases when the mother herself is hyperthyroid and is being treated with antithyroid drugs, the drugs end up treating the baby as well by crossing the placenta. However, if the mother's hyperthyroidism occurred in the past and was already treated with radioactive iodine or surgery, she can still have thyroid stimulating antibodies (TSAs) in her blood even though she's not hyperthyroid anymore. Since the mother is well and isn't exhibiting any hyperthyroid symptoms, fetal hyperthyroidism is simply not suspected. When the fetus is hyperthyroid, the fetal heart rate is consistently above the normal range of 160 to 180 beats per minute, and high levels of TSAs will be present in the mother's blood.

All women with Graves' disease or a history of Graves' disease should be tested for TSAs late in pregnancy. The consequences of untreated fetal hyperthyroidism can lead to low birth weight and small head size, fetal distress in labor, neonatal heart failure, and respiratory distress. Putting the mother on antithyroid drugs during pregnancy will treat the baby in this situation, but after delivery it will be necessary to continue treatment for the baby as well as performing follow-up tests.

Thyroid Disease in Newborns

Many people are confused by terms *neonatal* and *congenital,* which are sometimes used interchangeably. In medical terminology, neonatal refers to the first 28 days of life, while congenital simply means "present at birth."

Neonatal or Congenital Hypothyroidism

Neonatal hypothyroidism is different from congenital hypo-thyroidism. In the first case, the baby is born without a thyroid gland. In the second case, the baby is born with what appears to be a normal thyroid gland, but then develops symptoms of hypo-thyroidism after its first 28 days of life; this is known as *congenital hypothyroidism*, which is treated no differently than neonatal hypo-thyroidism. In this case, while the condition was present at birth, the symptoms didn't manifest until later. Congenital hypo-thyroidism is just as serious as neonatal hypothyroidism; symptoms may not be obvious until brain damage has already set in. The won-derful news is that neonatal screening for hypothyroidism in new-borns was introduced in the mid-1970s, and usually catches neonatal hypothyroidism while preventing congenital hypo-thyroidism from developing. Because growth and brain development are very dependent on thyroid hormone, this can be a very serious condition. If left untreated, the baby could be severely mentally re-tarded and suffer from growth and structural defects or dwarfism.

Neonatal hypothyroidism can also occur from an iodine defi-ciency in the mother's diet. This is common in more remote or mountainous areas of the world where iodine is not readily avail-able. In fact, iodine deficiency is the most common cause of mental retardation in underdeveloped countries. Fortunately, this is not a problem in North America, where all our table salt is iodized. (Low-salt diets still contain enough iodine for our needs.)

If hypothyroidism is diagnosed at birth, however, serious conse-quences are preventable by administering thyroid hormone replace-ment to the baby. In this case intellectual and physical growth will be normal. In North America all babies are given a heelpad test approxi-mately two days after birth to check for hypothyroidism; roughly one in 4,000 babies are born with neonatal hypothyroidism.

The heelpad test involves a blood sample that is taken by prick-ing the baby's heel and sent to a laboratory for analysis. Usually the test confirms that your baby's thyroid gland is functioning nor-mally. In rare instances the initial tests may be unclear, or inconclusive. If this happens, the laboratory usually notifies the hospital where your child was born as well your family physician. Someone will contact you to request another blood sample from your baby. If your child is in fact hypothyroid at birth, an endocrinologist and pediatrician will be consulted, and your baby will be placed on thyroid hormone replacement daily.

As a precaution, before you leave the hospital with your newborn, ask your doctor whether the heelpad test or thyroid test was administered. If for some reason the test was *not* done, request it, and make sure you find out the results of the test.

Neonatal Hyperthyroidism

Hyperthyroidism occurs only in infants born to mothers who are hyperthyroid. Most cases are not reported, and it occurs in one out of every 70 babies born to hyperthyroid mothers.

As discussed above, neonatal hyperthyroidism occurs when the fetal hyperthyroidism isn't caught. Fortunately, this type of hyperthyroidism in a newborn lasts only as long as the mother's antibodies remain in the baby's bloodstream, usually from three to twelve weeks. This condition is usually mild, since most women who are hyperthyroid produce only low levels of TSA.

Occasionally, if the hyperthyroidism is severe at birth, babies can be born with prominent eyes, irritability (more than usual), flushed skin, and a fast pulse—all classic hyperthyroid symptoms. These babies tend to be long and thin, and although they have large appetites, they may not gain any weight. The cranial bones also may be malformed. Some fetuses die before birth because of this illness, though. Infants who are hyperthyroid are always treated with antithyroid medication; radioactive iodine is never given to infants, and performing a thyroidectomy on an infant is unnecessary since the disease runs its course in 8 to 12 weeks. Sometimes *non*radioactive iodine (i.e., plain iodine) is used, however.

Thyroid Disease in Children

Congenital Goiter

There are several kinds of congenital goiters in children. In these cases thyroid function is usually normal and the only abnormality is a very large goiter. The treatment is to give thyroid hormone replacement, which causes the goiter to shrink by shutting down TSH production by the pituitary gland. Goiters are particularly common in girls around puberty, just as they begin to menstruate. As discussed in chapter 7, estrogen can often increase bound thyroxine levels in the blood (as opposed to active or free thyroxine), and estrogen levels peak just before girls begin to menstruate.

Sometimes a child's neck will look like a goiter is present, but in actuality the swelling is caused by an enlarged overlying fat pad, or by a growth of one or more lumps or nodules in the thyroid. You can recognize an enlarged fat pad if it doesn't move with your child's Adam's apple as he or she swallows. (Everyone has an Adam's apple; it simply enlarges in a male at puberty.) Enlarged fat pads are harmless. If nodules are present, make sure you get your child examined immediately in case the nodules turn out to be cancerous. As discussed in chapter 5, when thyroid nodules develop in children, they are statistically more likely to be cancerous than benign. Thyroid cancer in children is discussed later in this chapter. All children with swelling in the front of their necks should be examined by a doctor as soon as possible.

Hashimoto's Thyroiditis

The most common cause of goiters in children and teenagers is Hashimoto's disease. This usually occurs in children over six and in girls with a family history of thyroid disease. Aside from a goiter, there are usually no other signs of hypothyroidism unless the Hashimoto's disease is advanced. Hashimoto's disease is usually caught early in children because the goiter is an obvious sign that something is wrong. In children and teenagers, the treatment for Hashimoto's disease is the same as it is for adults: thyroid hormone replacement for life. When treatment begins, the goiter will shrink, but often the goiter is quite pronounced in children, so it may take a little longer to shrink. Generally, Hashimoto's thyroiditis in children does not cause any irreversible growth problems either physically or mentally. Undiagnosed hypothyroidism can certainly severely impede normal growth. But even in severe cases, growth resumes normally as soon as the child is treated, and any adverse effects caused by hypothyroidism are reversed.

One mother I interviewed told me that her perfectly healthy daughter suddenly stopped growing at the age of nine. Perplexed, she took the child to her pediatrician and was told that her daughter was simply going through a "phase." Unaware of thyroid disease and having no family history of thyroid problems, the mother accepted the pediatrician's diagnosis. After two years of stunted growth, this normally bright little girl started showing signs of incredible sluggishness and fatigue. She seemed to be unable to retain information and suffered from short-term memory loss. In addition, the child seemed unable to concentrate at all. She got extremely puffy (which is a classic symptom of myxedema, explained in chapter 2). Finally, after several second opinions, the mother was referred to an endocrinologist at a children's hospital. The endocrinolgist immediately diagnosed severe hypothyroidism and put the child on thyroid hormone replacement. Within days the child felt better, and although she was almost 12 years old by this point, she began to grow and develop normally. Today, she's perfectly healthy. This unusual story serves as a reminder that although hypothyroidism can severely affect a child's development, it is also a completely curable condition. The mother told me that she regarded thyroid hormone as a miracle drug.

Graves' Disease

Graves' disease also occurs in children, but it usually develops after the age of 12. Eye complications in children are rare, but they can happen. Usually, when Graves' disease occurs in a child, the child is extremely sensitive to the overproduction of thyroid hormone in his or her bloodstream. As a result, the child gets very sick quite quickly. Hyperthyroid symptoms can be obvious in children, as goiter or eye prominence are telltale signs. But often symptoms are more subtle, developing more slowly; irritability, for example, is difficult to catch. Things to watch out for are unusual tiredness (from exhaustion), a sudden growth spurt indicated by your child outgrowing clothing quickly, heat intolerance indicated by a child's sudden dislike for hot weather, or rapid fingernail growth. Classic adult symptoms such as palpitations and excessive sweating usually are not noticed by the child, but can be caught by a parent through day to day contact such as hugging, bathing, etc. If your child is involved with sports, weak shoulder and thigh muscles may be other signs to watch out for. Finally, if your child is unusually emotional (crying for no reason, for example), hyperthyroidism may be the culprit.

When children with Graves' disease get sick, the cause of their ailments is investigated as soon as possible. Thyroid function tests are often routine tests a pediatrician will run to try to find out what's wrong. Thyroid scans, however, are rarely done on children to prevent unnecessary exposure to radiation. When the diagnosis is made, treatment begins. Thyroid hormone levels are restored to normal, and the child will feel well again. Graves' disease in a child usually doesn't cause any permanent damage to normal growth and development (sometimes bone development is affected). If Graves' disease were to remain undiagnosed, the child may suffer some temporary problems that can be reversed with treatment. For example, any growth spurts that occurred as a result of hyperthyroidism will be offset by a long period of no growth. (If the child suffered from eye complications, he/she may endure permanent damage to vision in the long term.)

Treating Graves' disease in children is different than in adults, however. Antithyroid drugs are the first choice, since radioactive iodine isn't usually given to children or adolescents because their thyroid glands are more sensitive to radiation and are therefore more likely to develop tumors as a result of exposure to radiation. Usually, the hyperthyroidism is brought under control within a few weeks, but sometimes the child has to be on antithyroid medication for several months. Sometimes propanalol is used to slow down the heart. Some children have an allergic reaction to antithyroid medication, however. The allergy usually takes the form of a fever, hives, or a rash. One in 300 children on antithyroid medication develop a condition called agranulocytosis. Here, the child's white blood cell count is drastically lowered, which affects the child's immune system. If your child is on antithyroid medication, watch out for symptoms such as sore throat, mouth sores, and fever. If your child develops them, notify the child's doctor immediately and make sure the child is taken off antithyroid drugs at once. At this point, if the hyperthyroidism is still out of control, a thyroidectomy can be performed.

Sometimes, Graves' disease can be more severe in children than in adults. Because of this, antithyroid drugs often are not used at all, and the only route suggested is a thyroidectomy. After the thyroidectomy, if the child becomes hypothyroid, he or she will be placed on thyroid replacement for life. Although thyroidectomies are usually safe for children because children are smaller and more difficult to operate on, damage to the child's parathyroid glands, which control calcium levels, can occur. If this happens, the child may need to take calcium supplements for life. Another risk is accidental injury to the vocal cords, which could cause hoarseness. It should be stressed that these surgical slipups are rare, but sometimes doctors give parents the option of choosing radioactive iodine treatment instead.

Subacute Thyroiditis

Sometimes older children will develop an inflamed thyroid gland, usually an aftereffect of a viral infection of some sort. Your child will complain of typical common cold symptoms, but look for a goiter or a tenderness in the neck. This is a temporary condition that can be treated with aspirin or cortisone. See chapter 4 for more details.

Thyroid Cancer in Children

Many children are now being diagnosed with thyroid cancer, particularly in the aftermath of Chernobyl in Russia, Balarus, and the Ukraine. Radioactive fallout from both nuclear testing and nuclear reactor accidents are being identified as the culprits behind the increase worldwide (see chapters 6 and 11). Please pass on this section and other parts of this book to someone who can translate it if you have family members or friends in the Chernobyl aftermath who are dealing with a child's thyroid cancer. This information is just not available in these regions; and it should be.

Testing for Thyroid Cancer

As discussed in chapter 6, medullary thyroid cancer is a type of thyroid cancer that is inherited and passed down through the family. Although it's relatively uncommon, it still affects one in 50,000 North Americans. Recently, a new blood test can now screen for medullary thyroid cancer at birth. This blood test is not routine, but in families prone to this kind of thyroid cancer, a newborn can be tested for the gene associated with medullary thyroid cancer. This test is considered 99% accurate. The test was developed by a team at Barnes Hospital in St. Louis, Missouri, where various studies on medullary thyroid cancer were done. The team reports that on a study involving two families with a history of medullary thyroid cancer, 47 people in the families were tested for the cancer. Five of the adults were found to have already developed the cancer. Five of the children in the families were found to carry the gene that causes the cancer, which means that they are prone to developing the cancer when they grow up.

Generally, if anyone in your family has had this kind of thyroid cancer, you should request this blood test for your baby. If your baby tests positive, it doesn't mean your baby has thyroid cancer; it simply means the baby could develop thyroid cancer down the road. When the child enters his or her teens, he or she should be regularly screened for this type of cancer. As discussed in chapter 6, when caught early this form of cancer is almost always curable through surgery and radioactive iodine treatment.

When Your Child Is Diagnosed with Thyroid Cancer

As discussed in chapters 5 and 6, thyroid cancer is suspected when there's a hard, painless lump or nodule on or around your child's thyroid gland. Although some lumps in children are caused by thyroiditis or turn out to be benign cysts, when lumps are discovered around or on the thyroid of a child, they are more likely to be cancerous.

The investigative procedure of thyroid nodules in children is the same as for adults, and therefore radioactive iodine scans *are* used (see chapter 5). In this case the risk of thyroid cancer is considered greater than the potential risks of radioactive iodine. If the nodule turns out to be malignant, surgery followed by radioactive iodine is the treatment. Again, an exception to the "no radioactive iodine for children" rule is made because the risk of thyroid cancer is greater. In addition, in severe cases where the child's thyroid cancer is more advanced, external radiation therapy may be necessary. (Chapter 6 outlines thyroid cancer treatment in detail.) After treatment, your child will need to be on thyroid hormone replacement for life and will need to go for follow-up exams every three to six months for the first few years after treatment.

The most difficult part of the process is telling your child that he or she has thyroid cancer. Usually, the parent or guardian is notified by the child's doctor, and it's up to the parent or guardian to tell the child. As with any cancer, most children, if they're old enough, will be frightened by the word itself, but the worst thing you can do is lie to your child about the illness. All children vary in sophistication, but for most children under 10, the best way to break the news is to tell them that they need to have an operation on their thyroid gland. (For really young children, you can say that their thyroid gland is sick and needs an operation.) Then, gently prepare the child for what's ahead. You might want to explain the hospital trip as a sort of adventure so that the child won't panic when it's time to go. If your child has had his or her tonsils out in the past, you might refer to the thyroid operation as a similar experience (as long as the tonsillectomy was not a traumatic experience).

If the child is a preschooler, you could also use a play-therapy method of taking a favorite stuffed animal or doll and explaining that the animal or doll also needs an operation and will be accompanying the child to the hospital. You could cut a thyroid gland out of construction paper and paste it on the doll or animal, explaining to the child in simple terms how the animal or doll's thyroid works and that the thyroid needs an operation.

You'll probably take your child to a children's hospital for the surgery, or to the children's wing in a general hospital. These hospitals or wings are usually staffed with child social workers, child psychologists, or child care workers who will befriend your child and work with him or her to alleviate fears and answer questions. Your child will also have an opportunity to meet other children in the hospital, which is an excellent way to help reduce your child's feelings of isolation. Undoubtedly, many of the children your child will encounter in the hospital will be much sicker; they might have leukemia, cystic fibrosis, heart disease, kidney failure, AIDS, and so forth. Meeting these children will help your child realize how mild a thyroid operation is compared to the illnesses of other children.

Radioactive iodine treatment will also take place in the hospital. For young children (those under 10), you might explain the radioactive iodine as either a special pill or special water (depending on whether your child is given a capsule or liquid) that will make him or her better. Stress the fact that the pill or water doesn't hurt. To explain the isolation and precautions after the treatment, you can tell the child that in order for the special water or pill to work, he or she must follow very special instructions. You can then simply explain the various precautions and isolation procedures as "special instructions." Some parents/guardians may be tempted to use the word *magic* instead of *special* if they're dealing with very young children (for example, "magic pill" or "magic water"). This isn't a good idea.

It might confuse or distort the child's perceptions of what's real and what's fantasy. Furthermore, "special" is a much more truthful interpretation of radioactive iodine than "magic," which connotes sorcery rather than science. For older children or those interested in science, you can explain radioactive iodine in more scientific terms, and in fact educate the child about radioactive substances. (See chapter 11 for more details.) If you don't feel knowledgeable enough in this area, you and your child might look at some science books together that explain radioactivity, or ask your child's teacher to explain how it all works. You and your child's teacher could also supervise a special project in which the child can research radioactivity on his or her own, and explain radioactive iodine and radioactivity to the class.

If your child does have to have external radiation therapy, explain the radiation to young children as a special light or energy beam that will make him or her better. You must also prepare the child for the fact that the light/energy beam will cause the child to have a very sore throat. If the child has ever had tonsillitis or a tonsillectomy, explain the sore throat as a similar feeling to tonsillitis or having your tonsils out. Again, for older children or science buffs, a more scientific explanation is better.

For older and more mature children, treat them as you would an adult; try not to patronize them or treat them like babies. This doesn't mean that you have to come right out and say "You have cancer," but it *does* mean that you should tell them why they need to have an operation, what the procedure entails, and what kind of treatment they'll need afterward.

Children on Thyroid Hormone

Ultimately, whether your child is hypothyroid or hyperthyroid, or has been treated for thyroid cancer, thyroid hormone replacement for life is prescribed. Because they're continuously growing and developing, children on thyroid hormone will need to have their dosages monitored at least every six months and may require occasional adjustments. Often, family doctors or pediatricians will manage the child's thyroid dosage, but it's better to have your child referred to an endocrinologist before he or she reaches puberty. That way, any abnormality in sexual development because of too low or too high a dosage can be assessed and dealt with immediately. It's a good idea for girls on thyroid hormone to start seeing a gynecologist (in addition to an endocrinologist) when they begin to menstruate, so that any problems with their periods, mood swings, cycles, and so forth can be expertly dealt with.

For younger children on thyroid hormone, some of the play therapy methods described in the cancer section above can be applied here as well. For example, it's important that your child understands that he or she needs to take the thyroid pills every day to feel better. You can tell the child that thyroid pills are a kind of vitamin pill; for preschoolers, you can explain that a stuffed animal or doll needs to take the pills as well. Again, older children respond better with more scientific explanations.

For infants, toddlers, or younger children who can't swallow pills, you can crush the pill into their food. Unlike other pills, thyroid pills are not bitter; they have a sweet taste and therefore can be easily masked. In fact, thyroid pills also can be easily chewed and have the consistency of a chewable vitamin pill (although this is usually not directed on the label). Ask your doctor if your child can simply chew the pill instead of swallowing it. (This should be okay, but double-check!)

It's also important to teach your child to take responsibility for his or her own medication. To get your child in the habit of taking daily thyroid medication, you can get a pill box with slots for each day of the week. Or, have the child mark off on a calendar each day he or she takes the medication, so you can make sure that it's taken regularly.

In general, children with thyroid problems must understand that their condition, although cured, is permanent. For hypothyroid children, they must understand that as soon as they stop their medication, their thyroid problem will return; hyperthyroid children on antithyroid medication face the same consequence. Finally, hyperthyroid children or children with cancer whose thyroid glands were destroyed or removed must understand that they face hypothyroidism if they stop their medication.

Asking the Right Questions

As a parent, you're the one who can relay your child's symptoms to his or her doctor; you are the liaison between your child and doctor. You play a primary role in diagnosing thyroid disease in your child. The first step in preventing misdiagnosis is to make sure you report your complete family history to your child's doctor. If thyroid disease runs in your family, your doctor will pay extra attention to certain symptoms such as growth abnormalities.

Next, if you notice suspicious symptoms or signs, sit your child down and ask how he or she is *really* feeling. Here is a sample line of questioning:

1. I've noticed that you seem _____ (tired, emotional, and so on) lately. How are you feeling today?
2. Have you been sleeping okay? Are you having dreams? (Dreams indicate that the child reaches rapid eye movement [REM] in deep sleep. Sleeplessness is a sign of hyperthyroidism; too much sleep is a sign of hypothyroidism.)
3. When you wake up, are you still sleepy?
4. When was the last time you had a bowel movement?
5. What kind of bowel movement was it—mushy and soft, or hard? Light brown or dark brown? (This would help indicate diarrhea or constipation.)
6. Do you feel as though you're eating enough? Do you feel full or hungry after you eat dinner?
7. Do you feel cold at night, or too hot?
8. Have you been feeling sad, even though you have nothing to feel sad about?
9. Do you feel tired after you run around or play?
10. Do you notice your heart is beating fast sometimes?

These are some general questions that should confirm your suspicions. As I'll discuss in the next chapter, it's important to give your child's doctor as much information as possible to take the guesswork out of the diagnosis. The next chapter outlines how to make the best use of a doctor, whether it's your own doctor, your child's doctor, or an older parent's doctor.

A Layperson's Guide to Doctors

When you or someone in your family is diagnosed with a thyroid disorder, you usually wind up dealing with at least three doctors. Your family doctor is generally the first in a series of possible specialists, which can include an endocrinologist, ophthalmologist (for eye complications), head and neck surgeon, oncologist (a cancer specialist), radiotherapist, nuclear medicine specialist, nutritionist, dietitian, gerontologist (if you're older or are dealing with an older parent), and pediatrician (if it's your child). If your thyroid problem is misdiagnosed, you could end up seeing a psychiatrist, gynecologist, ear, nose and throat specialist, plastic surgeon (for nodules), heart specialist, internist, andrologist (male reproduction specialist), and a host of other specialists.

This is all very overwhelming. However, the most important relationship is the one you have with your family doctor. Whenever you're not well, it's your family doctor who sees you first and initiates the diagnostic process, which includes referrals to any one or a combination of specialists. The purpose of this chapter is to explain how doctor-patient relationships work in the 1990s, outline how to

make maximum use of your doctors, and minimize the frustration
caused by misdiagnosis.

How to Use a Family Physician

Since your family doctor is almost always the first doctor you'll see
about your thyroid problem, it's crucial that you understand the role
a family doctor plays in today's health care system as well as the role
a patient plays.

Keep in mind that your doctor is (a) only human and (b) running a business. Because medicine is a business, doctors are very
concerned about costs, so they try not to order too many tests or
unnecessary procedures. This can leave you misdiagnosed. As discussed in previous chapters, thyroid problems are often missed or
left undiagnosed by family practitioners until the symptoms become
obvious.

As a thyroid patient or potential thyroid patient, you have to be
responsible for making sure your doctor is acting in your best interests. To do this, you have to assert your rights as a patient and act re-
sponsibly at the same time. For example, if you keep certain
information about your medical history from your doctor, you can't
expect your doctor to make an accurate diagnosis. Similarly, if you
don't ask your doctor questions about your health, you can't expect
your doctor to answer the questions.

The Wrong Way to Use a Family Doctor

Here's a classic example of how a thyroid misdiagnosis occurs.
You're a 38-year-old woman with classic hypothyroid symptoms but
don't know it. You've noticed lately that you're not quite yourself.
You're tired, have no energy, and feel a little depressed. You decide
to go to your family doctor to let her know that you're not feeling
well and would like to know what's wrong. You arrive at her office.
As always, it's packed. She's overbooked again and you're after the

pregnant woman with three kids. Finally, she's ready to see you. You go into the examination room.

DOCTOR: *And how are we this morning?*
(TRANSLATION: The doctor wants to know if you're there for a checkup or have a particular problem.)

PATIENT: *You mean this afternoon.*
(TRANSLATION: You're letting the doctor know that you've been waiting a long time.)

DOCTOR: *Of course. Gosh, I've been so busy, I don't know where the morning has gone. Now what can I do for you today?*
(TRANSLATION: The doctor is telling you she's busy! She wants to know what your problem is—and make it fast because she has to fit in another 30 patients before 3 o'clock.)

PATIENT: *I've been feeling very tired the last few weeks and have almost no energy. I don't know what's wrong.*
(TRANSLATION: You're really saying that you feel rotten but can't prove it.)

DOCTOR: *I see. Any headaches, sore throat, stomach pains, nausea, vomiting, diarrhea, or unusual discharge?*
(TRANSLATION: Do you have a cold, flu, your period, or a sexually transmitted disease?)
PATIENT: *No.*

DOCTOR: *Let's have a look.*
(TRANSLATION: Do you have any idea how common these symptoms are? It could be anything! Give me a hint, at least!)

The doctor proceeds with the standard physical examination. You've said no to the discharge question, so that means that she won't do an internal.

DOCTOR:	*Well, everything seems to check out. Have you been under any unusual stress lately at work, or going through some problems at home?*
(TRANSLATION:	There's nothing apparently wrong with you. Your heart *is* a touch slow, but I don't think that's anything to be concerned about. I'm not saying anything. Why worry you more for no reason? It's probably just stress.)
PATIENT:	*No.*
(TRANSLATION:	I'm not imagining these symptoms. I'm here for a reason.)
DOCTOR:	*Have you been having regular bowel movements?*
(TRANSLATION:	What are your eating habits like?)
PATIENT:	*Now that you mention it, no. I have been constipated and I think I've put on some weight.*
(TRANSLATION:	You're kicking yourself for not saying this earlier, and you're worried the doctor isn't taking you seriously. She isn't. Should you also tell her you've been very sensitive to cold lately?)
DOCTOR:	*Periods regular?*
(TRANSLATION:	Do you have fibroids?)
PATIENT:	*Yes.*
DOCTOR:	*When was your last period?*
(TRANSLATION:	Are you pregnant?)
PATIENT:	*On the 15th.*
(TRANSLATION:	No, I'm *not* pregnant.)
DOCTOR:	*Tell you what, I'll order some blood work and call you*

if I see anything unusual. In the meantime, eat lots of fruits and greens, and try to get a little bran into your diet. A bran muffin for breakfast, for example. If you're still feeling the same a month from now, come back and see me.

(*TRANSLATION:* Maybe your diet's a bit off. I'll double-check your cholesterol and blood sugar just in case. Now go home. You're fine.)

The problem with this typical visit to the family doctor is that everyone's time was wasted. The patient gave the doctor very little information to work with, and as a result the doctor was only able to eliminate the problems. Although she did notice the slow pulse, it wasn't slow enough to alarm her. This patient will have to wait until her pulse is so slow that it's dangerous before the doctor connects it to a hypothyroid condition. In addition, the blood tests she ordered were standard. Tests that check TSH levels in the blood must be specifically ordered, so the doctor won't notice this thyroid problem for a while. (Although, in fairness, there are many family doctors who routinely check thyroid levels.) In the meantime, this 38-year-old hypothyroid woman will have to go home and get worse until the symptoms are bad enough for the doctor to put two and two together. And that can take a while.

In fact, the worst thing you can do is tell a doctor that you're tired and ask for a clear diagnosis. Family doctors report that the number-one complaint among their patients is fatigue. And it's a complaint that comes from people of all ages, occupations, and races. This woman needed more *facts* to be convincing in her complaint of ill health.

A major problem existed with the patient. She was clearly not very aware of her own body and wasn't paying enough attention to the signs. She noticed that she was tired and low in energy. That's a start, but it's not a lot to work with. Only when the doctor asked her about constipation did she remember. If she had reported all three symptoms at once, however, it might have prompted a different line of questioning.

The Right Way to Use a Family Doctor

When you notice something's off in your body—for example, if you're tired all the time—sit down and do a mental check of other things you're noticing so that you can give your doctor more than just tiredness to work with. Try to answer at least some of the following questions yourself:

Q: *Am I looking different than usual? How?*
A: I seem to have bags under my eyes that weren't there before and my hair's a bit drier. Come to think of it, I seem to have gained some weight as well.

Q: *Has my morning and evening bathroom routine (washing up and so on) changed at all? Am I going through certain skin and hair products faster than usual?*
A: I seem to be using more skin moisturizer than usual. I never did that before, and it seems like I'm always running low on hair conditioner. (This means your skin's drier and you're using more hair conditioner as a result.) Notice how this question confirms the observation in the preceding question about the dry hair.

Q: *Am I going to the bathroom more or less often than usual?*
A: Less. I've been constipated.

Q: *Am I eating any differently than usual to cause this, or trying to eat differently to remedy this situation?*
A: No. (So your constipation and weight gain are not linked to a change in diet.)

Q: *Am I feeling different than usual?*
A: I'm tired and I'm low in energy (also not linked to a change in diet).

Q: *Am I dressing differently than usual?*
A: I seem to always need a sweater now. I'm always cold.

Q: *Did my grandmother, mother, or father suffer from any kind of condition or ailment when they were around this age?*

A: I think Granny had a goiter after Mom was born, and Mom mentioned something about being on medication for her metabolism.

Q: *What is my pulse rate?* (If you normally check your pulse rate, find out if it's faster or slower than usual. For example, if your normal pulse rate is 80 and it checks out at 65 or 70, it's a bit low. If you don't know your normal pulse rate before you go to the doctor, phone your doctor's office and ask the receptionist/secretary to check your chart and tell you what your pulse rate was the last time you were there.)

Q: *Have I been under any unusual stress lately?*
A: No. (Now you can rule out stress-related symptoms.)

When you do it this way, you've taken a lot of the *routine* guesswork out of your doctor visit and may help the doctor get to the bottom of your symptoms faster. Let's replay that visit:

DOCTOR: *How are you this morning?*

Go for it! Don't hold back. Give her as much information as you possibly can. Symptoms run in groups, and you want to get the doctor to think about things that go together.

PATIENT: *I'm actually not that great. I haven't noticed any change in my daily routine—and I'm not under more stress—but I'm finding myself tired, low in energy, and constipated, and I think I've put on some weight, which is unusual for me. I've also noticed that my pulse seems a bit low. I'm usually at about 80 and it seems to be about five beats slower than normal. I don't know if this means anything, but I've also noticed that I seem to be cold all the time and that my skin and hair are dry. I know my grandmother had a goiter around my age and my mother mentioned something to me about being on medication for her metabolism. Do you think there's any connection?*

Wonderful. Any competent doctor at this point can rule out standard flu and cold symptoms and probably pregnancy. And that bit about the family at the end really helped. You haven't hit the nail on the head exactly, but this way the doctor is a lot warmer than in the first scenario. These kinds of symptoms still could involve some guesswork, but because you revealed what other members in your family were prone to, the doctor now has some idea of the kinds of conditions you're vulnerable to.

DOCTOR: *There could very well be a connection.*

From this point on, the doctor will probably ask more specific questions about your condition and try to get an even clearer picture. Every time you see her write something down on your chart, ask about it: What are you writing on my chart? Why is this or that significant? In other words, don't be afraid to challenge the doctor. Ask questions. If you don't understand something, keep asking until you do.

PATIENT: *What did you just write on my chart?*

DOCTOR: *I'm going to requisition some blood levels. I want to check your TSH.*

PATIENT: *What's TSH?*

DOCTOR: *Thyroid stimulating hormone—a secretion from your pituitary gland.*

PATIENT: *And what does all that mean? What do you think is wrong?*

DOCTOR: *You may have a thyroid condition.*

PATIENT: *Which means. . . .*

Depending on your doctor, he or she might get frustrated and try to end your questions. But don't stop. Remind the doctor who's in charge of your body. If things get really bad, ask him or her for some literature on the subject or a number you can call for more information.

| DOCTOR: | I'm afraid I'm running a little late. I don't have time to answer all these questions right now. |
| PATIENT: | I'm sorry, Doctor. It's just that it is my body, and I think I have the right to know what kind of tests you're scheduling and why. Can I make an appointment with you next week to discuss this in more detail? In the meantime, do you have any literature on the subject that I can read? |

Good. Now you're being assertive as well as sensitive to the doctor's schedule. Scheduling a separate appointment for questions is an excellent way to gain a better understanding of your health problem and a smart way to use your doctor's time. Asking for literature in the meantime indicates that you're willing to learn about your condition and participate in decisions.

Family doctors are used to treating a huge variety of illnesses and ailments within each age group. And they're also used to dealing with patients who range in medical awareness. In fact, a patient who actually takes an interest in his or her diagnosis is considered a rarity. And because a family doctor's scope is larger, it is naturally more general. Only within the last decade has the term *family practitioner* come to replace *general practitioner*. So the kind of response your questions are met with really varies.

However, if you have a doctor who is unwilling to answer your questions, you need to address the problem.

Keep in mind that much of the "right stuff" that makes a good family doctor is a combination of experience and instinct. The fact that they're human means that they do make mistakes, and the fact that they're businesspeople means that they're not risk-takers and may avoid unnecessary tests to cut costs.

The Patient's Bill of Rights

In the past doctors were expected to be godlike creatures while patients were expected to play very passive roles. This kind of doctor-patient relationship doesn't exist anymore. As patients, we're not only far more informed and sophisticated about health care than we were 20 years ago, but we are now also *consumers* of health care. We've gone from patient to *im*patient. We want results; we want value for our money. Whether we live in the United States or Canada, the patient is the one who pays the doctor's salary. (Canadians pay for health care through their taxes.) As a result, the doctor-patient relationship is now a two-way street—not unlike a marriage. What do you have a right to expect from a doctor?

1. *As much information as you want.* This means that you have every right to know your diagnosis, prognosis (your doctor's estimate of when you'll get better), alternate forms of treatment, your doctor's recommendations, and the basis of his or her recommendations (research studies, hunches, and so forth).
2. *Time to address questions and concerns.* If your doctor doesn't have time to answer questions, you should be able to call him or her or make another appointment that serves as a question-and-answer period.
3. *Reasonable access.* You and your doctor must decide together what "reasonable" means. Do you need weekly, quarterly, or annual appointments, or do you just want to see the doctor when you feel like it? How much advance booking time do you need to get an appointment?
4. *To participate in the decision-making process.* To do this, you'll have to ask questions and be willing to educate yourself about your illness (such as requesting literature on your illness from your doctor).
5. *Adequate emergency care and to meet your doctor's substitute.* Who looks after you after hours when your doctor's sick or on vacation? Is there a substitute doctor? You'd better find out in case you need to see the substitute someday.
6. *To know who has access to your health records.* How confidential are your health records? Can your doctor release them to just anyone—your employer, insurance companies, government authorities? What are your doctor's legal obligations with respect to health records, and what are *yours*?

7. ***To know what it costs.*** If you live in the United States, you have the right to know what your bill is in advance. Get an estimate and have the doctor break down each charge so you know exactly what you're paying for and what your insurance plan is covering. If you live in Canada, make sure all appointments, tests, and procedures are covered by your province before you consent to anything.
8. ***To be seen on time.*** If you're on time for an appointment, your doctor should be as well. Do you generally have to wait more than 30 minutes in the reception area before your doctor will see you? (Obviously, there are going to be times when a doctor is going to be called away on emergency or needs to spend more time than anticipated with a particular patient.)
9. ***To change doctors.*** Yes, you can fire your doctor. If you're unhappy with your current doctor or simply need a change, you have every right to switch. Make sure you arrange for your records to be transferred!
10. ***A second opinion or a consultation with a specialist.*** If your doctor can't make an adequate diagnosis, you can insist on a referral to either another doctor or a specialist.

The Doctor's Bill of Rights

Remember, it's a two-way street. Your doctor has an unwritten bill of rights, too. Just as you're entitled to certain information and courtesies, so is your doctor. So what exactly does your doctor have the right to expect from *you*?

1. ***Full disclosure.*** Doctors aren't telepathic. If you're hiding information (certain family or medical history, prescriptions, addictions, allergies, eating disorders, specific symptoms) it's unfair to expect an accurate diagnosis. What if your doctor prescribes a drug that you're allergic to, for example, or one that conflicts with other medication?
2. ***Common courtesy.*** Treat your doctor like a business associate. If

you make an appointment, show up; if you need to cancel, give 24 hours' notice.

3. *Advance planning.* Plan your visit in advance, and think carefully about your symptoms. Don't just go to your doctor with a vague complaint like "I'm not feeling well" and expect a full diagnosis. When you make an appointment, tell the receptionist how much time you think you'll need for a full examination, and write down your symptoms. Give the doctor something to work with.

4. *Questions and interruptions.* If you don't understand something, ask. Interrupt the doctor if necessary, and ask for simpler explanations of what's wrong. If you don't do this, you can't blame your doctor for not giving you enough information.

5. *Follow advice and follow through.* Take medication as directed and follow advice. That's what you're paying the doctor for. If you're experiencing side effects to medication, have a problem with his or her advice, or your condition has worsened as a result of the doctor's advice, let the doctor know. Full disclosure strikes again.

6. *No harassment.* If you have a problem, go through reasonable channels; dial the after-hours emergency number the doctor leaves with the answering service, or call your doctor's office during business hours. Don't continuously call the doctor at home at 4 o'clock in the morning, and don't call the office 10 times a day with every little ache and pain.

7. *Enough time to make a diagnosis.* Diagnoses don't happen overnight. Allow the doctor enough time to examine you, run necessary tests, and so forth. Don't expect miracles in 15 minutes. This may mean that you will need to wait longer for an appointment so your doctor can schedule enough time to fully examine you.

8. *Room for disagreement.* What you think is in your best interests may not be what your doctor thinks is best. Allow for a difference of opinion and give your doctor a chance to explain his or her side. Don't just leave in a huff and threaten to sue. Maybe your doctor is right.

9. *Professional conduct.* Don't request unusual favors that compromise your doctor's moral beliefs, and don't ask your doctor to do

something illegal (for example, writing bogus notes to your employer so you can claim disability pay).

Incidentally, if even a few of these rights are abused, your doctor has the right to resign as your doctor and request that you seek care elsewhere.

Guidelines for Choosing a Family Doctor

If you have the luxury to choose any doctor you wish, or if you are on an insurance plan that offers you a wide selection of doctors, here are some general guidelines.

Family doctors, by tradition, treat the entire family and therefore develop an intimacy with each particular family member and familiarity with family health problems. Today, the family doctor's role has changed significantly in that the doctor often has no connection with the health scenario in your family. If you're in this situation, make sure your doctor is aware of not just your own history, but your *family's* medical history.

However, you can encounter problems with a doctor who has in fact treated your whole family. Again, it does depend on the doctor, but if you're a woman, often the worst thing to do is to go to your mother's doctor after you're 18. The doctor may continue to treat you as a child and may discuss your health situation with your parent(s), bypassing you in the process.

A doctor who delivered you may be an uncomfortable choice for internal examinations or breast exams. Sometimes it's important to make that break. If you're between 20 and 35 and uncomfortable with a doctor you've seen since childhood, you can ask him or her to recommend a good family doctor. If you're afraid of offending the doctor, ask him or her to recommend a gynecologist—you should have one anyway—and then ask the gynecologist to recommend a family doctor. Of course, if you *are* comfortable with the same doctor who has treated your mother and father, then *don't* switch, but make a point of evaluating your doctor. You may want to even see a few other doctors just to see who's out there.

If you're a woman between the ages of 39 and 55, you should also reevaluate your situation. Menopause is a very sensitive time, and the worst thing is to have a doctor who is insensitive to you. What may have worked for you in your late twenties and early thirties may not work anymore. If loyalty's an issue, forget it. If you are not comfortable with your doctor, you will avoid going, and in the process endanger your own health.

If you're older, try not to take your doctor's word as gospel. The older you are, the more abused you can become in the process. You're given less information, you're often not treated as equally as someone closer to the doctor's age, and if English is not your first language, you may be easily intimidated.

No matter how old you are, if you don't speak English well, you're at an immediate disadvantage. It's very important to find a doctor who speaks *your* language. If you speak Cantonese, so should your doctor. If you speak Greek, your doctor should as well. If you can't find one who does, call an association or organization affiliated with your ethnic origin and ask them.

Women doctors versus men doctors? That depends on you. If you're a woman who is more comfortable going to another woman, or a man who is more comfortable with a man, do it. Men and women often feel better with a doctor of the opposite sex. But follow your preference. The most important question is whether you're comfortable with your doctor. It's shocking how many people aren't.

Here is a quick checklist you can use to evaluate how comfortable you are with your *current* doctor:

1. *What does your doctor call you?* Your doctor should call you by the name you're most comfortable with—be it your surname, first name, or nickname.
2. *How old is your doctor?* Your doctor should ideally be within about 15 years of your own age. That way he or she is your peer, not your father/mother or son/daughter. This makes it easier to relate to your doctor.
3. *Can you ask your doctor questions?* How open is he or she? If you can't question your doctor, that's a bad sign.

4. *Where is your doctor located?* Is the location convenient, or does it take you over an hour to get to? Waiting to see the doctor is stressful enough, but if you're hiking across the country just to go to your doctor, consider the stress involved with your doctor appointments.

5. *Can you reach your doctor by phone?* Can you just pick up the phone and call him or her anytime to talk about a particular health situation? If you can't, is it because the doctor is truly busy or just not accessible after hours to patients? Some doctors, for example, leave an emergency number where they can be reached.

6. *If he or she weren't your doctor, would you want him or her as a friend?* If you wouldn't be caught dead having a cup of coffee with your doctor, why would you take off your clothes in front of him or her?

7. *Does your doctor make house calls?* If he or she does, you probably *do* have a gem on your hands.

Finally, keep in mind that family practitioners are not specialists and therefore have very different temperaments and expectations from their patients. A family practitioner usually chooses family medicine over other specialties because he or she likes the contact with the public, the intimacy with the patient, and the variety in general. While there are a few who practice family medicine because they're sick of residency and don't have the energy it takes to become a neurosurgeon, all of them are human beings and you're bound to find someone you can relate to.

When to Get a Second Opinion

Getting a second opinion means that you see two separate doctors about the same set of symptoms. The doctors can be in the same field or specialize in different areas. This can happen at either the diagnostic or treatment stage of an illness. Second opinions often come into play in the diagnosis and treatment of various thyroid disorders and illnesses. Often, the doctor will want you to see one of his associates or a specialist to confirm a diagnosis or a particular treatment approach; this is known as a consultation. Sometimes the patient requests a referral to another family doctor or specialist to seek an alternate diagnosis or approach to treatment; this is what we've come to know as a second opinion, although a consultation is the same thing.

Second opinions can be tricky, however. There are a variety of factors doctors weigh in determining the best treatment. For example, a 30-year-old, single woman with Graves' disease may be prescribed antithyroid drugs by one doctor, while another doctor may want to use radioactive iodine. In the first case, perhaps the doctor wishes to spare risking radioactive iodine, since the woman is in prime childbearing years; he may not want to risk radioactive iodine just in case the woman is in the very early stages of pregnancy, or feel that the woman's anxiety over the long-term effects of the treatment may do more damage. In the second case, the doctor may feel that radioactive iodine, a speedier and more results-oriented therapy, will treat the illness once and for all; after all, prolonging the illness will prolong the woman's suffering, and radioactive iodine is perfectly safe as long as the woman is not pregnant. Both approaches are right, but it is the woman who will choose the treatment she's most comfortable with. Yet the same doctor who wishes to use antithyroid medication on this woman may want to use radioactive iodine on another Graves' disease patient, a woman with four children who is divorced and 40 years old.

Second opinions can be lifesavers, particularly when a thyroid disorder is misdiagnosed. For example, misdiagnosed Graves' disease symptoms are often caught by eye specialists—ophthalmologists. In these cases patients may go to their family doctors and complain of some general hyperthyroid symptoms that imitate stress symptoms. They are told to slow down and come back if the symptoms persist. Not connecting their sudden eye problems to these more general symptoms, Graves' patients often seek out referrals to an ophthalmologist regarding their sudden blurred vision or pain in their eyes. At this point it is the ophthalmologist who would diagnose exophthalmus (eye bulging), a condition caused by thyroid disease, and then refer the patient to an endocrinologist.

A 50-year-old woman with classic hyperthyroid symptoms that include missed periods may be diagnosed by her family doctor as having menopausal symptoms and may be prescribed estrogen hormone supplements. (Not an outrageous diagnosis given the woman's age and symptoms.) In this case the woman would be wise to request a referral to a hormone specialist—an endocrinologist—who would take a variety of blood tests to check the woman's hormone levels before he or she prescribed anything. Thyroid levels in this case would probably be routinely checked, and the woman's problem would be caught here.

Finally, let's take my own experience as a second-opinion case in point. When I was 20, I noticed a hard, painless lump in my neck, and I went to my family doctor. At first, my family doctor didn't think the lump was serious and assured me that millions of people develop benign cysts every year; it was probably nothing. He told me to come back in a month if the lump was still there. A month later the lump hadn't changed and I went back. At this point, my family doctor referred me to a plastic surgeon because plastic surgeons are good at assessing normal tissue from abnormal tissue. In this case my doctor didn't feel qualified enough to make this assessment and sent me on his own recognizance for a second opinion. The plastic surgeon, on a hunch, felt that a biopsy of the lump should be done, and I had a lumpectomy. At that point, the lump was found to be malignant and was traced to my thyroid gland. I was then referred to a head and neck surgeon, since I would require surgery. However, had my family doctor told me to go home and not worry about the lump, I might have done so. We tend to seek second opinions when there's bad news; but when the doctor tells us what we want to hear, we don't want to tempt fate. Incidentally, this same family doctor had diagnosed my mother with Graves' disease only a couple of years earlier; when he saw me after the lumpectomy, and after my thyroid cancer was diagnosed, he asked me to tilt my head back and felt my thyroid gland. The gland was clearly enlarged. My doctor then said with frustration: "I don't know *how* I could have missed that!" In other words, even though my doctor had full knowledge of my family history, and my thyroid gland was visibly enlarged, the lump was still not an obvious giveaway. Accurate diagnoses are difficult, and doctors are fallible. What made him a good doctor in this scenario is the fact that he recognized his own fallibility and sent me for a second opinion.

Guidelines for Seeking a Second Opinion

It's difficult to know whether you're justified in getting a second opinion. For example, just because you don't like the sound of your diagnosis doesn't mean you require another opinion. For example, let's say you have an obvious goiter, classic hyperthyroid symptoms, and bulgy eyes; your doctor wants to perform a radioactive iodine uptake test to confirm his or her suspicions. You might not like the sound of this and decide to see a holistic doctor or a herbalist instead. This person may tell you that you're under stress and only need to rest and adjust your diet. Of course, this is a much more calming diagnosis, but your medical doctor is the one who is right.

The following is a set of guidelines that should help you decide whether a second opinion is warranted. If you answer yes to even one of the questions below, you're probably justified in seeking a second opinion.

1. *Is the diagnosis uncertain?* If your doctor can't find out what's wrong or isn't sure whether he or she is correct, you have every right to go elsewhere.
2. *Is the diagnosis life-threatening?* In this case, hearing the same news from someone else may help you cope better with your illness or come to terms with the diagnosis. Diagnoses like cancer, however, usually won't change; the diagnosis is based on carefully analyzed test results, not just the patient's symptoms.
3. *Is the treatment controversial, experimental, or risky?* You might not question the diagnosis but have problems with the recommended treatment. For example, if you're not comfortable

with radioactive iodine, perhaps another doctor can recommend antithyroid drugs or surgery.

4. *Is the treatment not working?* If you're not getting better, maybe the wrong diagnosis was made or the treatment recommended is just not for you. Occasionally, antithyroid medication doesn't work, and radioactive iodine turns out to be the best approach after all. In this case, seeing someone else may help to clear up the problem.

5. *Are risky tests or procedures being recommended?* If you don't like the sound of a radioactive iodine scan, hearing it from someone else might make you accept the procedure more readily. Perhaps a blood test or biopsy is a better route for you. Find out if there are alternate procedures that can confirm the same results.

6. *Do you want another approach?* An 80-year-old woman with heart disease and high blood pressure might be diagnosed with thyroid cancer. She'll probably die from heart disease or a stroke before she dies from thyroid cancer, which grows very slowly. As a result, her doctor may decide that she's too frail for surgery and treatment and opt to leave her alone. The woman's children may find this approach unacceptable and demand that her thyroid cancer be treated.

7. *Is the doctor competent?* When I asked my gynecologist if radioactive iodine treatment would conflict with the Pill, his response was "What's radioactive iodine?" I left and never went back. I eventually found an excellent gynecologist who was well versed in thyroid disease and cancer. Basically, if your doctor doesn't seem to know very much about other health problems you have and doesn't bother to find out, go somewhere else! Or, if you only suspect your doctor is humbug, go somewhere else to reaffirm your faith in him or her or confirm your original suspicions.

Doctors Say the Darndest Things

I was convinced this section should be added when I recently received a call from a young woman who had been treated for thyroid cancer. She was put on thyroid hormone replacement at too high a dosage (this happens) and became severely hyperthyroid as a result.

Her doctor's response was, "You're *supposed* to be hyperthyroid after cancer treatment or else the cancer can grow back." No attempt was made to lower the dosage, perform blood tests, or even prescribe beta blockers. When this woman phoned me, her pulse was over 200 beats per minute, and she had lost more than 15 pounds. I asked who her doctor was, wanting to know who could mismanage her so badly.

She replied, "It's my endocrinologist. He's the only one in town."

"Well does this doctor treat thyroid disease or mostly diabetes?"

"Mostly diabetes."

I gave this woman the number of a thyroid foundation chapter in her area, which had lists of *thyroidologists,* a term used to describe endocrinologists who specialize *solely* in managing thyroid disease. I told her that it was worth getting on a bus, train, or plane to get the right specialist. I then explained to her that, while, yes, thyroid cancer patients need to be on a higher dosage of thyroid hormone pills in order to totally suppress their TSH, it was absolutely *not necessary for these patients to ever experience hyperthyroid symptoms.* My TSH has been suppressed since 1984, and I have never experienced even moderate hyperthyroid symptoms as a result. This woman also phoned me in tears because her family doctor told her radioactive iodine causes leukemia, at which point I explained that radioactive iodine does not cause leukemia, breast cancer, or any other kind of cancer.

The point is that just because your doctor has a medical degree, doesn't make him or her a thyroid specialist. If something doesn't sound right, it may not be. Please contact either me (care of my publisher) or any of the organizations listed at the back of this book to check it out.

Here's a case in point from my own medical history. After a routine check up with my family doctor, she called me to say that my T$_4$ readings were a little high, and she felt that I would be better off on a slightly lower dosage. I told her that I would check with my endocrinologist, who manages my thyroid condition. My endocrinologist, however, informed me that my family doctor's instincts were appropriate for someone who has a history of thyroid disease, *not* thyroid cancer. In fact, my TSH needs to be suppressed, which is why my T$_4$ readings were slightly high. So again, a medical degree doesn't automatically mean "thyroid specialist."

A dozen ways to be mismanaged

Here are 12 of the most common errors primary care doctors make when diagnosing or managing a thyroid condition.

1. Many don't know very much about radioactive iodine therapy. Therefore, a lot of misinformation and just plain *wrong* information gets out to the patient. You may be told that you can never have children, or that your risk of leukemia triples. All of this is wrong, wrong, wrong. See "The Long Half-Life of Radioactive Myths" in chapter 11 for more information.
2. Many insist that you don't need to see a specialist. This is not appropriate. Many primary care doctors don't know what they don't know. You should always have your thyroid problem *first* assessed by a specialist. Indeed, your thyroid disorder may not be complicated, and may be easily managed by a primary care doctor, but don't assume so until you hear from a thyroid specialist.
3. If you're lucky enough to be referred to an endocrinologist for a thyroid problem, many primary care doctors don't realize that not all endocrinologists are thyroid specialists. Many treat strictly diabetes and only "dabble" in thyroid, as demonstrated in the anecdote above. See the section on how to find a thyroid specialist for more information. Worse, many diabetes specialists don't know what they don't know about thyroid disease!
4. Many still tell you your symptoms are stress-related or diet-related.
5. Many ignore lumps in the neck and tell you "it's nothing." Never ignore a lump anywhere on your body. Get a second, third, or fourth opinion, if necessary, before you dismiss it.
6. If you're a woman, many doctors will still tell you that your symptoms are related to PMS, menopause, chronic fatigue syndrome, and even chronic yeast of all things! (I hear this often.)

7. Many will refer you to a psychiatrist mistaking your symptoms for biological depression. Or, you'll be referred to a variety of wrong specialists.

8. Some mistake Hashimoto's disease for thyroid cancer, because of the firmness of the goiter. So, instead of a TSH test and an antithyroid antibody test, you have a fine needle biopsy and a thyroid scan!

9. Many fail to recognize a TSH deficiency, which means that on top of your hypothyroidism, you'll experience problems with your reproductive glands (often pubic hair falls out) and adrenal glands. Symptoms range from complete loss of libido to blood sugar problems and high blood pressure. This can send you bouncing from one specialist to another for months.

10. Most fail to distinguish between thyroid problems and aging. A classic problem is the failure to diagnose what's called *apathetic hyperthyroidism,* which affects seniors. This means that you'll have slight hyperthyroidism but not severe enough to be obvious. You may have just a slight increase in pulse, slight loss of energy, and so on. Seniors represent the most under diagnosed group of thyroid patients in the world.

11. Some doctors still prescribe thyroid hormone replacement to perfectly healthy women for weight control. This is almost criminal and warrants a medical malpractice suit. As I say in chapters 1, 2, 12, and 13, thyroid problems are not the cause of a weight problem once the thyroid problem is treated. Thyroid hormone replacement is not a weight loss drug and is only intended as treatment for hypothyroidism and other thyroid problems. A healthy person taking this medication will eventually die of heart failure. Weight problems after a thyroid problem is treated are caused by the usual: lack of exercise combined with the wrong diet. See the "Nutrition for Eu" section in chapter 13 for more information on low fat and healthy eating.

12. Many primary care doctors are behind the times when it comes to thyroid testing and order obsolete blood tests that measure bound and "inactive" thyroid hormone instead of "free" and active hormone. As discussed in chapter 2, the appropriate tests

are TSH and FT_4 (free T_4). TT_4 (total T_4) is obsolete, but if it's being done, you need to have a T_3 resin uptake test, as well.

How to Use a Specialist

Specialists are a different breed from family physicians. They're more academic: They teach or run residency programs, they're involved with research, they frequently lecture at various academic centers, they regularly publish papers, articles, and books in their field, and they're recognized in their field. Specialists train longer than family doctors, make more money (internists and endocrinologists make only slightly more, though), and charge more for their services. As a result, many specialists are more egotistical, colder in terms of bedside manner, harder to get in touch with (they're usually booked months in advance), and because they're pressed for time, impatient. Certainly there are many specialists who are very caring and do not fit this profile, but don't be surprised when you find one that *does!*

In addition, you usually don't have the luxury of shopping for a specialist the way you do for a family doctor, because you're only referred to one when you need one. At that point your main concern is getting better as soon as possible, and "getting in" to see another specialist can take months—time you really can't afford when you're ill.

Again, you have rights, and specialists, like any other doctors, have their rights as well. Because their time is valuable (not to mention expensive), here are some guidelines to follow that will help you make maximum use of your specialist:

1. *Tape record your visit.* Specialists often say a lot in a small space of time. When you're upset or overwhelmed by all of the information being hurled at you, you often don't hear what the specialist is saying. Tape recording the visit is helpful because you can replay information when you're more relaxed, and thus better understand what you've been told.

2. *Take a list of questions with you and tape record the answers.* When you have a lot of questions, make a list so you don't forget them. The specialist has an obligation to answer all of your questions, and if he or she doesn't have time, there are some options. Give him or her your list and ask if he or she can address them in your next appointment. If that's not possible, agree on a time when the specialist can call you at home and address the questions. As a final resort, ask if there is a resident studying with the specialist with whom you can arrange a question-and-answer session. (Usually, any resident, a specialist-in-training, can address your questions.)
3. *Request literature or videos on your illness from the specialist, or get the number of an organization that you can call for more information.* In my case, many of the specialists I saw were flattered that I found "their work"—my body—so interesting. If they have more information about your illness, they'll usually be happy to share it with you.
4. *If it's relevant, ask the specialist to draw you a diagram of your illness.* My head and neck surgeon actually drew me a diagram of the thyroid, carefully explaining where my cancer was.

How to Find a Thyroid Specialist

This can be tricky, as many of my readers have told me. First, not all endocrinologists "do" thyroid. Many solely specialize in diabetes, or even *reproductive* endocrinology. Thankfully, many solely specialize in thyroid disorders, too. Second, if you need thyroid surgery, not all general surgeons do thyroid surgery, while endocrinologists do not do thyroid surgery. And, if you live in a small community where there is one endocrinologist serving the whole population (this is common, and they often know more about diabetes than thyroid), then your search will be challenging. Here's the shortest route to a good thyroid specialist (it's not foolproof, though):

1. Call a thyroid organization at the back of this book for a list of

thyroidologists—and use that term—in your area. If the person on the other end of the phone says, "Huh?" say "endocrinologists who specifically specialize in treating thyroid disease."

2. Go to your primary doctor and ask to be referred to at least two specific names on that list. (Many health plans require a referral to specialists.)

3. Make an appointment with *both* doctors so you can interview them. Ask them how many thyroid cases they manage each year. If the answer is under 10, and I'm being generous, that specialist doesn't see many thyroid patients. Then, ask how many diabetes patients that specialist sees per year. If the number is disproportionately higher, you may be in the wrong office. Also ask how many fertility patients that specialist sees per year (just to make sure you don't end up with a fertility specialist or a reproductive endocrinologist).

4. If you're still unsuccessful, ask people you know if they know someone with a thyroid problem. And then, call them. Who are *they* seeing? You may need to go outside your area to a larger city, but it's worth the trip to avoid being mismanaged, which will cost you more in the long run.

5. Once you're with a thyroidologist, that doctor will manage the rest of the referrals to ophthalmologists (for thyroid eye disease), head and neck surgeons (for surgery), nuclear medicine specialists (for radioactive iodine therapy), oncologists (for thyroid cancer), and so on. See the next section for a glossary of terms.

Map to the Specialists

Since it's a little difficult to hunt for a thyroidologist when you don't know if you need one, you may encounter at least three different specialists for your thyroid condition. The first doctor is usually a family doctor, the doctor who will initiate the referral or consultation process. The following is a map to some of the specialists you'll encounter, including a brief description of when you'll be referred to each one.

Endocrinologist: This is a hormone specialist or, more precisely, a doctor who specializes in the endocrine system. Since the thyroid produces a hormone, an endocrinologist will understand all of the complexities involved with thyroid hormone. If you're hypothyroid or hyperthyroid for *any* reason, you'll be referred to an endocrinologist. Generally, endocrinologists will manage your thyroid hormone replacement dosage and will supervise any other form of treatment, including radioactive iodine therapy or thyroidectomy.

Ophthalmologist: This is an eye specialist, someone you'll only encounter if you're having eye problems as a result of Graves' or Hashimoto's disease. Either your family doctor or endocrinologist will refer you to one.

Cardiologist: If your hyperthyroidism is causing palpitations or a heart slow-down, your endocrinologist or family doctor might send you to this person.

Head and neck surgeon: Generally, your endocrinologist will call in a head and neck surgeon (under the endocrinologist's supervision) if you need to have a thyroidectomy. For example, if you have a particularly wicked case of Graves' disease and are in a situation or age group where you can't have radioactive iodine, surgery may be the route to go. If you have a nasty goiter that isn't responding to thyroid hormone, surgery also may be necessary. If you have thyroid cancer, however, surgery is always necessary. In this case, often it is the family doctor who refers you directly to a head and neck surgeon, bypassing the endocrinologist altogether.

Nuclear medicine specialist: If you need radioactive iodine you'll briefly visit the nuclear medicine department and encounter a specialist in nuclear medicine who will explain how radioactive iodine works and go through the scan or treatment procedure with you. This is a one-night-stand sort of relationship. Your endocrinologist or head and neck surgeon routinely consults with this department for your treatment, but your care is never transferred to the nuclear medicine department.

Radiation oncologist: If you have thyroid cancer and need external radiation therapy, either your head and neck surgeon or endocrinologist will send you to a radiotherapist (a doctor who specializes in external radiation therapy) who will manage the radiation portion of your treatment.

Oncologist: This is a cancer specialist, whom you'll encounter if you have thyroid cancer. Sometimes head and neck surgeons are also oncologists.

Pediatrician: If your child has a thyroid problem and you don't already have a pediatrician, you'll be referred to one by a family doctor, obstetrician (if the problem is discovered at birth), or endocrinologist.

Gerontologist: This is a doctor who specializes in diseases of the elderly. If you have an older parent who has a thyroid problem, a gerontologist may be called in as a consultant. Sometimes it is the gerontologist who calls in an endocrinologist.

Gynecologist: If you're female and have a thyroid problem, seek out a gynecologist on your own, or ask your endocrinologist or family doctor to refer you to one. (You should have one anyway!)

Andrologist: This is a doctor who specializes in male reproduction. Sometimes, men with thyroid problems experience sexual problems or fertility problems. If this is the case, an endocrinologist may refer you to one of these.

Ear, nose, and throat specialist: Also known as an ENT, you might end up with this specialist if your family doctor is baffled by various thyroid symptoms (for example, thyroiditis, lumps in the throat area, and so forth).

Psychiatrist: When your family doctor tells you your thyroid symptoms are either stress-related or "just your imagination," you'll be sent to a psychiatrist.

Gastroenterologist: This is a G.I., or gastrointestinal, specialist. You may be sent to one if you have symptoms of heartburn, bloating, and constipation.

Of course, there are a few other specialists on the thyroid *mis*diagnosis trail that I haven't bothered to map. Basically, the purpose of this chapter is to acquaint you with the business of medicine 1990 style. The old rules are gone. Patient accountability and responsibility are paving the way for healthier doctor-patient relationships. That means requesting more information and becoming educated about your illness. The next chapter is the one to read if you've had or will have radioactive iodine scans or treatment.

A Layperson's Guide to Radioactive Iodine

The most frightening aspect of radioactive iodine is that it's a very complicated substance to both explain and understand. One must be acquainted with atomic physics and biology to fully comprehend its positive medicinal use on the one hand and its negative risks on the other hand.

In fact, unless a doctor specializes in nuclear medicine or frequently consults with other nuclear medicine specialists, he or she may not have the background to give you a satisfactory explanation of what radioactive iodine actually is. That's why it's important either to question directly the doctor who is administering the radioactive iodine to you, or to call a reliable source, such as the one listed below, for the most up-to-date information.

What is Radioactive Iodine?

You don't have to be a nuclear physicist to understand radioactive iodine. (But it helps!) Charmingly known as the "atomic cocktail," radioactive iodine was discovered accidentally in the 1940s as a by-product of research carried out at the atomic laboratory in Oak Ridge, Tennessee. Although it sounds pretty scary, it's simply the unstable form of iodine.

The development of nuclear medicine, used to diagnose and treat certain thyroid disorders, is based on the use of radioactive elements and particles for both testing and treatment. *Radioactive* is the adjective used to describe elements containing *unstable atoms*, or atoms that are emitting energy and hence releasing radiation. A radioactive element is called an isotope, meaning "unstable element."

Imagine, for example, that you're trying to carry 300 loose ping-pong balls in your arms from one end of a room to the other without dropping any. It's impossible. Inevitably, as you try to balance and juggle the balls, some *will* drop and fall from your grip. This is essentially what happens when an element like iodine is radioactive.

The iodine atoms can't securely grip the particles in their center. As a result, some of these subatomic particles "fall." The element is therefore unstable. But unlike the ping-pong balls, when these particles, or energy (particles *are* energy, incidentally), hit the "ground"—in this case, living tissue cells—they can damage and mutate the cells.

This is why exposure to too many radioactive particles can cause violent sickness and cancer (like what happened to the victims of Hiroshima and Chernobyl). However, if you are being treated for cancer, radiation and radioactive particles can be used in a positive way. In this case the goal of the treatment is to damage your mutant cancer cells deliberately and prevent them from reproducing and spreading throughout your body. To treat various thyroid diseases and thyroid cancer, radioactive *iodine* is used because the thyroid naturally absorbs this particular element.

Testing

As you now know, radioactive iodine is used in thyroid testing and as the standard form of treatment given exclusively to patients who are hyperthyroid from diseases like Graves' or who are diagnosed with thyroid cancer. But it's also used as a tracer for certain diagnostic tests.

The Uptake Test: Testing Function

As mentioned in previous chapters, doctors will occasionally want to explore thyroid function further through the radioactive iodine uptake test. It determines how hungry the thyroid is for iodine, which can explain the cause of hyperthyroidism, and provide more information about nodules, cancer, and goiters. The thyroid's iodine appetite may be affected by many factors aside from thyroid function alone. (Blood tests such as the free T_4 test and the TSH test, discussed in chapter 2, are still the most accurate for determining thyroid function.) Abnormality is determined by reading how much radioactive iodine is absorbed by the thyroid. This is either a 4- or 24-hour test, depending on the tracer used.

When you arrive at the hospital, you're given a minuscule amount of radioactive iodine. It may be in the form of a capsule or waterlike liquid. You ingest the iodine and go home. You are usually (but not always) given some sort of instruction pamphlet that tells you how to reduce the risk of radiation exposure to others around you, even though there is no risk involved with a small tracer dose.

There is more than one isotope or recipe of radioactive iodine available, but isotopes with an atomic weight of either 123 or 131 (usually referred to I^{123} or I^{131}) are the ones most widely used. There is currently a debate within the nuclear medicine community as to whether I^{123}, which allows you to be scanned at only two hours, is more effective than I^{131}, which requires 24 hours before you can be scanned; some physicians believe that I^{123} subjects patients to less radiation but does the same job as I^{131}. At any rate, the test is known as the I^{131} uptake test. The next day, you return to the hospital and sit in front of a huge, cameralike instrument. A conelike device is brought up to your neck area and the machine then measures the amount of radioactive iodine absorbed by your thyroid. This instrument is known as a scintillation, or counting probe.

If your hyperthyroidism is caused by an overproduction of

thyroid hormone, your uptake, or absorption, of the radioactive iodine is high (usually more than 30% in 24 hours). Since there are other reasons for an elevated uptake, this test is combined with other diagnostic procedures to obtain an accurate diagnosis. If you are hyperthyroid but your uptake is low, your hyperthyroidism is probably caused by either an overdose of thyroid hormone replacement or by some sort of inflammation in the thyroid.

If you are hypothyroid, this test is often useless. It doesn't allow this kind of diagnosis to be made, and to diagnose hypothyroidism, a blood test is required. So it is not commonly used.

The Imaging Test: Testing Structure

The basic difference between an uptake test and an imaging test is that the uptake test measures thyroid performance while the imaging test measures form. The thyroid imaging (scanning) test is similar to the uptake test and is used to check thyroid structure. Also a 24-hour test, the purpose of an imaging test is to check the size of a large goiter or to check for hot or cold nodules, described in chapter 5.

An imaging test is also done to check the success of a thyroidectomy procedure, verifying how much (if any) thyroid tissue is still left in your body. Again, you are given a tracer of radioactive iodine (I^{131} or I^{123}), or technetium. Usually a slightly higher dosage is required for this test. When you return to the hospital the next day, you lie down under a large camera or imager (the scanner) that takes pictures of your thyroid. The iodine absorption is visible from the pictures taken, and your doctor can tell by the images how much structural damage exists. Sometimes a body scan is necessary if thyroid cancer is present. The only difference between a body scan and a thyroid scan is that the imager takes pictures of your entire body to make sure that the cancer hasn't spread beyond your thyroid.

If you're being given this test as a follow-up to a thyroidectomy (usually only performed in the event of thyroid cancer), your doctor will take you off your thyroid hormone replacement. This is done to induce a hypothyroid state deliberately and trigger the release of TSH into your blood. TSH will stimulate the cancerous tissue to absorb iodine and the test becomes far more accurate. The same thing is also done if you're being treated for thyroid cancer.

Depending on your condition and the hospital, something called TC pertechnetate, a more convenient tracer, is used instead of I^{131} or I^{123} for both the uptake and imaging tests. When TC pertechnetate is used, your thyroid is exposed to only one one-hundredth of the radiation that would occur with I^{123}, for example, and the tests can be performed only 20 minutes after this tracer is administered. This is probably the new wave of radioactive iodine, and by the year 2000 both I^{131} and I^{123} may very well be regarded as a medical anachronism for diagnostic testing.

Treatment

Radioactive iodine used for treating hyperthyroidism and thyroid cancer, however, is still very much in vogue and has been for some 40 years.

Hyperthyroidism

In cases such as Graves' disease, radioactive iodine is used to destroy enough of the gland to cure the hyperthyroidism. Although it is ideal to damage just enough of the gland to bring the patient back to a normal level, a by-product of this treatment may well be hypothyroidism, because it's difficult to determine a precise dose that will not destroy too much of the thyroid. It's a feast-or-famine situation. This is very easily remedied, though. If the gland isn't able to produce a normal amount of thyroid hormone, you're immediately put on thyroid hormone replacement (to be taken daily) to bring you back to the euthyroid, or normal, state.

The treatment for Graves' disease is similar to the first stage of the diagnostic tests described earlier, only you're given a far more potent dose of radioactive iodine. Until recently, a curie, named after Marie Curie, is the unit of measurement used for radioactive substances. Doses of radioactive iodine were given in either milli-curies (one-thousandth of a curie) or microcuries (one-millionth of a curie). The term now coming into use is *megabecquerel* (after Henri Becquerel, who discovered radioactivity).

A typical dose of radioactive iodine for treatment of Graves' disease would consist of anything between 3 and 12 millicuries (or 100 to 500 megabecquerels), while a radioactive iodine tracer for an uptake test would consist of anything between 4 and 6 microcuries. A tracer for an imaging test (or scan) would range between 30 to 100 microcuries. A dosage over 30 millicuries requires hospitalization, but dosages in treatment for Graves' disease only occasionally reach such potency. You're usually sent home immediately after treatment, but depending on your dosage, you might have to observe the rules outlined below to avoid exposing others around you to the radiation you received.

For hyperthyroidism, a single dosage is usually required to do the trick. It's usually painless, regardless of whether you're given a capsule or liquid. Only in very high dosages (over 30 millicuries) would you feel any discomfort. With a higher dosage, you might feel some tenderness in your neck. Sometimes a high dosage affects the saliva glands, causing your mouth to feel dry after the treatment. But that's really all. You're rechecked (through a blood test usually) at six weeks, three months, nine months, and then annually. Radioactive iodine does not go to work immediately on your hyperthyroidism. Your symptoms are not going to disappear overnight. It takes at least four to six weeks, and often closer to three months for the treatment to decrease the size of your thyroid gland and thyroid hormone secretion. Fifteen percent of all patients treated with radioactive iodine for hyperthyroidism will need a second dose, while 5% may even need a third helping. Ultimately, 20% of people receiving this treatment for hyperthyroidism will become hypothyroid (a sign that you're cured), and then will need to be on thyroid hormone replacement for life to return to a normal thyroid state. Generally, 50% of all people treated with radioactive iodine can expect to be hypothyroid in 10 years. That's why its very important to have regular thyroid function tests every six months or so.

Thyroid Cancer

As discussed in chapter 6, radioactive iodine treatment for thyroid cancer involves a very high dosage that ranges between 100 and 150 millicuries. Again, this dosage is only given if the cancer was discovered in a *secondary* stage; when detected earlier, enough thyroid cancer may be treated through surgical means only.

After a high dose of radioactive iodine (over 30 millicuries) you're kept in isolation in a private hospital room for at least two days and are not permitted any visitors. There's usually no discomfort, other than the effects mentioned above with high dosages. When you're released from the hospital, you'll then be required to practice the precautions listed below. (Chapter 6 outlines radioactive iodine treatment and posttreatment precautions for thyroid cancer in detail.) After about 10 days, you may need to undergo one more imaging test to make sure that the treatment *worked*—it almost always does—and then you're usually home free.

Posttreatment Precautions for Regular Dosages

Depending on your doctor and hospital, after you've received an average treatment dose of radioactive iodine, you may need to follow some hygiene precautions for the next two or three days. The reason for such precautions is to prevent the exposure of radiation to others through your saliva, sweat, mucus, urine, feces, or other bodily secretions. It's a good idea to drink an extra two to three eight-ounce glasses of water during this period; it helps you "pee out" the excess radioactivity faster. It's a lonely couple of days, but it's necessary. In the worst case scenario, if people were exposed accidentally, they wouldn't get sick, but they'd be exposed to an unnecessary level of radiation that could cause some harm to their healthy thyroid glands. The dosage for Graves' disease usually has a half-life of about eight days. That means that in eight days, the radiation is half as potent as it was when it was first administered. After about two or three days, the remaining radioactive particles in your body deteriorate considerably, and you're no longer a "threat" to anyone around you.

In fact, the amount of radioactivity in your system becomes quite negligible at this point. For the first few days, the main things to keep in mind are to reduce closeness and contact with others, and keeping yourself very clean.

You'll need to minimize contact with pregnant women or small children, because children, infants, and fetuses are more sensitive to radiation exposure. Use different or disposable dishes and cutlery, and wash them separately. Abstain from all sexual activity (including kissing), sleep alone, and wash your linens separately after use. You should use a separate hairbrush, comb, towel, and face cloth, and wash out the sink or bathtub after each use. After you use the toilet, wash your hands carefully, flush the toilet about three times after use, and use separate toilet paper. If you use the telephone, you must wipe the mouthpiece with a damp cloth after use. You should separately launder everything you wear or use. Drink a lot of liquid to help the radioactive iodine pass through your urine faster.

With most treatment doses for Graves' disease and tracer doses for scans, which fall under 30 millicuries, there isn't any *medical* need to follow these precautions. But some hospitals or clinics may ask you to observe the precautions anyway—regardless of your dosage—because of certain institutional regulations. For higher dosages (over 30 millicuries), you would need to be isolated legally for 48 hours. But most doctors feel the radioactive treatment dose for Graves' disease is so low, the above precautions are *not* necessary. Again, it depends on your doctor.

Notes for Women

If you're a woman in your childbearing years, a pregnancy test is typically required because you *must not* be given radioactive iodine therapy if you're pregnant. The radioactive iodine can injure the thyroid gland of the developing fetus. If you're not asked to take a pregnancy test, demand one, even if you're on the Pill or are regularly menstruating. It's very important that you don't take a chance. Sometimes, even after a negative pregnancy test, you can still discover that you're pregnant. (Usually, tests don't pick up the pregnancy until about six weeks.) If you've had the radioactive iodine treatment and then discover you're pregnant, your obstetrician may want to perform a therapeutic abortion. This depends on the circumstances. If you're in the very early stages of pregnancy, the thyroid gland doesn't develop in the fetus until the twelfth week, so you're still considered safe. If you're planning to become pregnant, check with your doctor and find out how long you have to wait before you can conceive. Usually it's about six months.

If you're breast-feeding, you must stop after you have radioactive iodine because it passes through your milk to your baby. Check with your doctor to find out when you can start again. Usually, waiting about three months after the treatment is acceptable. See chapter 7 for more details. For more information on pregnancy or breast-feeding, consult my books, *The Pregnancy Sourcebook* and *The Breast-feeding Sourcebook*.

How to Get Information

Believe it or not, sometimes patients aren't given any kind of material or pamphlet on either the treatment itself or these precautions. If you're not given any literature on this at the time of your treatment, ask your doctor about these precautions, or call one of the organizations at the back of this book.

The Long Half-Life of Radioactive Myths

After talking to hundreds of thyroid patients around the continent, this treatment has been the source of a huge number of myths that have a pretty long half-life. Here are some of the most common myths that I wish to dispel, once and for all.

MYTH: *Radioactive iodine causes leukemia.*
FACT: Wrong! Even if you had something like 500 millicuries of radioactive iodine (Graves' patients get anything from 4 to 30 millicuries, while thyroid cancer patients get 100 to 150), only about 5 out of 1,000 people on that dosage would go on

to develop leukemia, which could not be *absolutely* linked to the radioactive iodine. So, even in this super-exaggerated circumstance, your chances of developing leukemia are 0.5%.

MYTH: *Radioactive iodine causes breast cancer.*

FACT: People who have undergone radioactive iodine therapy, including myself, have the same chance as anyone else of developing breast cancer. Right now, we don't really know what causes breast cancer, but there is no increased incidence of the disease in people who have had radioactive iodine. For more information on breast cancer risk, consult my book *The Breast Sourcebook*.

MYTH: *Radioactive iodine causes other kinds of cancer.*

FACT: This isn't true, either. Your chances of getting a particular kind of cancer have to do with your family history and genetic makeup. None of this is altered by radioactive iodine.

MYTH: *Radioactive iodine causes birth defects.*

FACT: This is only true if you have the treatment while you're pregnant, which wouldn't happen because no competent doctor in his or her right mind would ever recommend this treatment to a pregnant woman. As long as you wait six months after this treatment before trying to conceive, you will be fine. (Of course, pregnancy carries other risks which have nothing to do with radioactive iodine.) See "Notes for Women" on page 188 and chapter 7 for more information, and on pregnancy risks, consult my book, *The Pregnancy Sourcebook*.

MYTH: *Radioactive iodine causes your hair to fall out.*

FACT: Wrong! People say this because they are confusing this treatment with external radiation therapy, which also does not cause hair loss unless the scalp is radiated. People may also be confusing this treatment with chemotherapy, which often causes hair loss.

MYTH: *People with seafood allergies cannot have radioactive iodine therapy.*

FACT: While seafood contains iodine, the allergy to seafood is rarely a reaction to iodine. So, people with this allergy usually do fine. The amount of iodine in an average radioactive dose for Graves' disease amounts to less than 1 microgram anyway. But if you're concerned, see an allergist beforehand.

MYTH: *When hypothyroidism sets in after treatment, you've had an overdose of radioactive iodine.*

FACT: The point of radioactive iodine therapy is to ablate or destroy the thyroid gland and turn it into a dried-up raisin. This will eliminate your hyperthyroidism permanently. So, if you're *hypo*thyroid after this treatment, *good*! That means it worked, and you don't have to repeat the therapy. To restore thyroid hormone, all you need to do is take a pill, something I discuss at great length in the next chapter. Some doctors enjoy the challenge of giving you just the right amount of radioactive iodine to cure the hyperthyroidism, without making you hypothyroid. This is a hotly-debated issue right now. Many doctors feel this approach is fruitless, due to the nature of autoimmune thyroid disease. For most cases of Graves' disease, the thyroid gland will continue to overproduce thyroid hormone no matter how precise a radioactive dosage you have. You can't have a normal thyroid with Graves' disease any more than you can be "sort of" pregnant. Treatment for thyroid cancer has different goals, discussed in chapter 6.

How Radioactive Iodine Affects Healthy Thyroid Glands

I've included the following information for thyroid patients, their families, and their friends because I strongly believe that understanding both the positive and negative sides of radioactive iodine alleviates fears associated with radioactive iodine treatment. Let's face it, the precautions are frightening. Worse, when you're given radioactive iodine out of a lead container from someone who is wearing protective gloves, and told that "it's perfectly safe" but to "stay away from your children," you're not exactly put at ease. Obviously, the lead container, the protective gloves, and the precautions are in place for a reason—to protect people with healthy thyroid glands. But thyroid patients receiving radioactive iodine in its medicinal form are not the only sources of risk to a healthy thyroid gland.

As nations around the world become more industrialized and energy efficient, they are also becoming more nuclear smart. Ironically, although the threat of global nuclear war has diminished, the threat of nuclear reactor accidents is still very real; radioactive iodine can be emitted in the fallout of reactor accidents—it happened at Chernobyl. So understanding radioactive iodine is useful not only for people who are receiving radioactive iodine scans or treatment, but for anyone with a healthy thyroid gland as well.

Understanding Chernobyl

One of the first indications of the accident at Chernobyl in 1986 was the detection of radioactive iodine (I^{131}) and other radioactive isotopes in countries near Russia. If radioactivity escapes during a nuclear reactor accident, it is usually in the form of small amounts of radioactive gases. Chernobyl was different. Here, the reactor core overheated and large amounts of radioactivity escaped from the melted fuel pellets. Because iodine vaporizes easily, *radioactive* iodine was released and was carried high into the atmosphere for long distances by air currents. This radioactive material then settled to the ground as fallout.

Obviously, breathing in radioactive iodine fallout is a concern for people with normal, healthy thyroid glands. So what are the implications and consequences of an accident such as Chernobyl?

In this kind of accident, the air can expose people far away from the accident to radiation via a fallout cloud of radioactive iodine I^{131}. This isotope has a half-life of eight days and therefore can exist for several weeks before it breaks down or decays. Other radioactive iodine isotopes have shorter half-lives which consist of minutes or hours and simply don't last long enough to travel a significant distance. When these isotopes are released in reactor accidents like Chernobyl, they're generally heavier and fall to the ground sooner. So the air in this case is only a problem for people living in the immediate vicinity of the reactor. But this creates another problem.

When these radioactive iodine particles fall on plants that may be food for man or animals, there is a risk of ingesting radioactive iodine fallout. For example, if cows graze in areas that are contaminated with radioactive iodine, the radioactivity that enters the cow's system can be secreted in the cow's milk. If people drink this milk, the radioactive iodine will then enter their bodies. Similarly, if people eat fallout-contaminated food, the radioactive iodine can enter their bodies directly.

Since the thyroid gland normally absorbs iodine to function, each thyroid hormone molecule contains three or four iodine atoms—T_3 and T_4. But since the thyroid can't distinguish between radioactive iodine atoms and normal iodine atoms, both will be collected in the thyroid gland and synthesized into thyroid hormones that will circulate in the blood.

As long as the thyroid gland is working normally, it will absorb a proportion of the radioactive iodine it's exposed to.

If an individual is given a large amount of normal iodine in the form of potassium iodide before or during the exposure, the normal iodine will saturate the thyroid gland and prevent it from absorbing the radioactive version. In other words, by ingesting large quantities of regular iodine, the thyroid gland becomes "full," and simply "can't eat another bite" of either normal or radioactive iodine. As a result, any radioactive iodine that is absorbed will be excreted through the body in its urine. It's important to note that radioactive iodine is only dangerous to a healthy thyroid gland; it cannot cause any other kind of cancer such as leukemia, for example. (Although chapter 7 discusses how a woman's breasts also trap iodine, radioactive iodine is not known to pose any danger to breasts, nor is it known to have ever caused breast cancer.)

The Children of Chernobyl

The nuclear accident at the Chernobyl atomic power station, on April 26, 1986, exposed millions of people with healthy thyroid glands to excessive levels of radioactive iodine. People living within a 30 kilometer zone of the accident inhaled the radioactive iodine, while people living outside the 30 kilometer zone ingested the radioactive iodine. For reasons not quite understood, potassium iodide was not distributed to any of these people. Now, there appears to be a *twenty-fold* increase in the incidence of thyroid cancer in children in Belarus, Russia, and the Ukraine. For example, in one study out of the Ukraine, between 1981 and 1985, the number of new cases of thyroid cancer in children ages 0 to 14 totaled 25. But between 1986 and 1994, the number of new cases of thyroid cancer in this age group totaled 210, with peak periods in 1992 and 1993.

While children's thyroid glands are sensitive, it's important to note that children exposed in utero seem to represent a large number of new thyroid cancer cases. Ninety-five percent of all thyroid cancer in Chernobyl children is papillary cancer (see chapter 6). This is treated the same way as it is in North America: total thyroidectomy followed, ironically, by radioactive iodine.

There aren't many agencies looking out for these children, but there is an organization in Toronto, Canada that specifically helps to fund these children. For more information about what you can do to help as a fellow thyroid sufferer, contact the Children of Chernobyl Canadian Fund, listed in the resource section at the back of this book. Clothing is particularly appreciated, but if you know of someone in that area who is affected, please pass on information you receive from organizations, or passages of this book. If possible, have sections translated. There are very few support structures in place for the frightened families and children affected by this disaster.

Potassium Iodide: A Blocking Agent

Since potassium iodide can prevent radioactive iodine from being absorbed by the thyroid gland, it's known as a thyroid blocking agent. However, it can only protect against radioactive iodine; potassium iodide has no protective effect against any other kind of radiation. In fact, pharmacists report that when the Persian Gulf War broke out, large quantities of potassium iodide were dispensed to people who lived in communities with nuclear reactors. In some cases doctors were prescribing it, in other cases people were requesting potassium iodide tablets on their own.

In general, doctors are reluctant to use potassium iodide to protect the thyroid, however, unless it is "really necessary." To be effective, the potassium iodide must be given just prior to being exposed to radioactive iodine and then continued for the duration of the exposure. This is pretty difficult to do unless an accident is predicted in advance, or the air path of a specific accident is tracked and therefore anticipated.

Practicality is another problem; it's simply not smart to continue to administer potassium iodide over longer periods of time. The main reason is because potassium iodide can have some significant side effects over long-term use. Complications range from a variety of serious allergic reactions and skin rashes to thyroid disorders (like hyperthyroidism). The thyroid problems potassium iodide can trigger can be particularly trying for people who have autoimmune diseases like Graves' or Hashimoto's. In these cases, potassium iodide may trigger sudden hypo- or hyperthyroidism. In pregnant women, potassium iodide can also cause the fetus to develop a goiter.

Finally, potassium iodide will have no effect as a blocking agent on people whose thyroid glands have been surgically removed or who are already taking thyroid hormone replacement tablets of some kind. However, in these circumstances radioactive iodine would not be a problem because it wouldn't be absorbed by the thyroid; the thyroid would either be gone or not functioning.

What If You Are Exposed to Radioactive Iodine Fallout?

If you think you've been exposed to radioactive iodine, make sure you do what I call a thyroid self-exam, or TSE. Every couple of months, look in the mirror and visually inspect your neck area for signs of a goiter or unusual lumps and bumps. Put your head back as well to get a better look at your thyroid area. Hard lumps are especially suspicious, particularly if they are under your ear lobe or further around your neck area. Then, feel your entire neck area from the nape at the back all the way around. If you find a lump, request that a fine needle aspiration be done to rule out cancer. See chapters 5 and 6 for more information on other possible signs of thyroid cancer. You won't find information on how to perform a TSE in the same way you might for breast self-exam. This is a term I've coined, but one I hope will catch on in the thyroid world.

When to Take Potassium Iodide

For the last 30 years, various government agencies around the world have monitored the amount of radioactive iodine in the air. For many years they have detected low levels of radioactive iodine fallout as a result of nuclear testing carried out across the globe (most recently by China and France). If serious reactor problems are anticipated or actually experienced, the authorities would order the immediate distribution of potassium iodide to people who might be exposed. In North America, for example, almost all of the reactors have advanced safety features and effective containment devices to prevent the release of radioactive gases.

The Three Mile Island accident was the most serious reactor accident to have occurred in North America, but the average population exposure from radioactive iodine in that accident was very small— much less radiation than a chest X ray, and thousands of times less than a routine diagnostic I^{131} uptake test. Because of these facts, and the possible effects of radioactive iodine, both the American and Canadian food and drug administrations have not released potassium iodide as a drug for thyroid blocking, except to state/province and local governments who stockpile it for emergency use.

Although inadvertent exposure to radioactive iodine is something that should be guarded against, it's important to remember that radioactive iodine is perfectly safe for people with thyroid disorders! There have been a series of careful follow-up studies done on patients who received radioactive iodine since the 1950s. So far, the studies conclude that it is perfectly safe. Thyroid patients who receive radioactive iodine treatment go on to lead healthy, productive lives, suffering no ill- or aftereffects from the treatment.

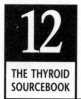

Thyroid Medication

When you're taking thyroid medication, you're either on thyroid hormone replacement for life to compensate for a hypothyroid condition (often the result of treatment for hyperthyroidism), or you're taking antithyroid medication to control hyperthyroidism. Depending on your condition, age, sex, weight, and lifestyle habits, your doctor will recommend one of these two forms of medications. This chapter covers common concerns thyroid patients have about their medication and also outlines other substances or drugs thyroid medications can conflict with. The pharmacist-patient relationship is also discussed, an issue that concerns anyone on lifelong medication.

Thyroid Hormone Replacement

Thyroid hormone has come a long way. In the 1890s, medical textbooks provided recipes for preparing animal thyroid glands as a treatment for thyroid patients. You were likely to have fried, minced thyroid, served with bread and currant jelly for breakfast. A few decades back, the form of thyroid hormone replacement used was desiccated thyroid hormone, which was composed of dried animal thyroid hormone. Unlike the synthetic hormone today, dried animal thyroid hormone was a mixture of T_4 and T_3, and no two mixtures of desiccated thyroid hormone were alike. For example, one pill may have contained three parts T_3 and one part T_4, while another contained the reverse. As a result, although desiccated thyroid hormone worked, it was jarring to other bodily systems since the levels of T_3 and T_4 always varied. Because of this, it also had a shorter shelf life. (It is still considered a perfectly good medication, however.) Worse, many people who had their thyroids removed through surgery prior to 1960 were often not prescribed desiccated thyroid hormone; many family doctors felt their patients "didn't need it" (as was the case with my grandmother, who had a goiter removed in 1940). Fortunately, doctors are far more sophisticated about thyroid hormone, and desiccated thyroid hormone isn't used anymore because of the availability of much higher quality synthetically produced thyroid hormone replacement pills. A prescription for thyroid hormone replacement pills costs anything from $15 to $30 for a three-month supply, depending on the brand.

Thyroid hormone replacement pills are color coded. This is done to improve what pharmacists refer to as patient compliance. When each dosage comes in a different color, its much easier for patients to say "I'm taking the pink pill" rather than "112 micrograms," for example. See Table 12-1 for a complete list of colors, dosage strengths, and suggested guidelines according to weight. These thyroid pills, as we patients call them, are simply a replacement to what your body normally produces. Therefore, allergic reactions or any other side effects are very uncommon. Most people can take thyroid hormone replacement tablets without worrying about side effects and lead a perfectly normal existence.

On one hand, when you're on thyroid hormone, there are also no special diets to follow, nor will you have to restrict your routine in any way. On the other hand, you will have to get into the habit of taking medication at the same time every day. In order for your body to function as if it were producing thyroid hormone normally, you must supply it with the replacement hormone regularly. For hypothyroidism, the average dose is roughly around 112 micrograms. Most people will be able to find the right dose for themselves in the seven or eight dosage strengths between the 50 and 150 micrograms range. The average daily dose after thyroid cancer treatment ranges from 100 to 200 micrograms. Please see "Note for Thyroid Cancer Patients" below for more information.

Rarely patients can be allergic to some of the dyes used in synthetic thyroid hormones. This can cause upset stomach, gas, nausea, and muscle aches. Your doctor can usually prescribe synthetic thyroid hormone without the dye. Most brands offer their 50 microgram strength as a plain white pill, without dye. Pharmaceutical manufacturers recommend that you ask your doctor to prescribe your thyroid hormone replacement in increments of the white pill (such as 50 micrograms) if you're experiencing a reaction. See "What's in This Stuff?" further on for more information.

If you're on too high a dosage of synthetic thyroid hormone, you'll develop all the classic symptoms of hyperthyroidism. If this happens, notify your doctor; he or she will adjust your dosage accordingly. The correct dosage of thyroid hormone is determined by a normal TSH reading, (0.5 to 5 mU/L). A reading greater than 5 mU/L suggests that you're hypothyroid, while a reading less than 0.5 mU/L suggests that you're hyperthyroid. T_4 readings may also be checked. The normal range is between 50 and 165 nmol/L, but most people feel best when the readings are above 110. However, you should never stop taking thyroid hormone or alter your dose (taking two pills per day instead of just one) without consulting your doctor. It's also important to make sure you tell any other doctor you're seeing (such as various specialists or a new family doctor) that you're on thyroid hormone. Thyroid hormone replacement can affect the potency of certain prescription and nonprescription drugs. If all of your doctors are aware that you're on thyroid hormone, potential problems can be avoided if they need to prescribe other medications.

Note for Thyroid Cancer Patients

The appropriate thyroid hormone replacement dosage is slightly different for thyroid cancer patients. That's because the goals of therapy are a little different, as well. Any microscopic piece of thyroid tissue in your body will be stimulated by TSH. If that thyroid tissue is cancerous, then TSH may stimulate cancerous tissue to grow. In this case, the trick is to find a high enough dosage to suppress your TSH, which means that your T₄ readings will be *higher* than those of plain old hypothyroid patients. But you need not suffer any hyperthyroid symptoms. TSH suppression can be accomplished with one of the precise doses offered by brand-name thyroid hormone replacement pills. Common dosages for thyroid cancer patients are 125 or 137 micrograms (137 micrograms is not available in Canada). The appropriate range for TSH suppression is anywhere from 100 to 200 micrograms.

Appropriate Dosages for Children

As discussed in chapter 9, children are certainly not immune to either thyroid disease or thyroid cancer. The recommended daily dose for children taking thyroid hormone is 5 to 6 micrograms per kilogram of body weight for babies ages 0 to 12 months old; 3 to 5 micrograms per kilogram of body weight for preschoolers 1 to 5 years; 4 to 5 micrograms per kilogram of body weight for children age 6 to 10 years; and for children over 10, the appropriate dose goes by adult body weight, indicated in Table 12-1. The rule here is 1.6 micrograms for every kilogram of body weight.

If You're Elderly or Have Heart Disease

To avoid any risk of being overreplaced (i.e., overdosed to the point where you're hyperthyroid), dosages of thyroid hormone should start fairly low at around 12.5 micrograms (a 25 microgram pill cut in half with a special pill cutter is available in all pharmacies). Dosages should be adjusted very, very slowly, in increments of 25 micrograms until you reach the right thyroid levels.

Generic Versus Brand-Name Hormones

Synthetic thyroid hormone replacement is one of the most popular products pharmacists dispense. In the United States, more than 15 million prescriptions of thyroid hormone per year are sold annually. Even if only part of your thyroid gland was surgically removed, thyroid hormone replacement may be prescribed. A large pharmacy will order the pill by the thousands and could easily dispense a thousand pills per week (that's 10 prescriptions for 100 pills). It's also not unusual for pharmacists to come across 100 pills with 12 repeats, which is about four years' worth of pills. Because of the demand, there are a variety of drug manufacturers that make thyroid hormone medication, so it can be purchased as a brand-name or generic product. The generic thyroid hormone, universally known as levothyroxine, (aka L-thyroxine) is cheaper, but the quality control on generic products may not be as strict as it is for brand-name products. This is particularly important for older patients who depend on a precise dose. In light of this, it's probably best to always request a brand-name thyroid hormone replacement product such as Synthroid, Levoxyl, or Levothroid. The brand names are all equally good, though.

The key phrase in a quality thyroid hormone replacement pill is precise dosing. This enables your doctor to prescribe the lowest, most effective dose without overdoing it, or underdoing it. It's also important to keep in mind that thyroid hormone brands are not interchangeable. Endocrinologists have seen definite variations in thyroid function after patients have switched brands. The right dose for you on Brand A may not be the right dose for you on Brand B. So, the shortest route to maintaining thyroid hormone function with your thyroid pill is to:

1. Choose a quality, name-brand thyroid hormone pill that offers *precise dosing*. (Table 12-1.) This is particularly important for women over 40, who may be approaching menopause; anyone over 60; as well as people with heart conditions. If your doctor tells you that generic preparations are just as good (as my own primary care doctor once told me), this is just *not* true.
2. Stay on the same brand; don't switch around. Again, since you may require a different dose on Brand A than you do on Brand B, just stay on the brand you're on.

Table 12-1
The United Colors of Thyroid Hormone Replacement Pills

Thyroid hormone replacement is color coded by dose. Dose is usually determined by weight, unless the goal is TSH suppression, or there are other medical conditions at work. Below is a *general* guideline only, in micrograms, assuming approximately 1.6 micrograms of thyroid hormone replacement daily for every kilogram of adult body weight. After 65, expect your dosage to decrease by about 10%. Eltroxin is available only in Canada. Levoxyl and Levothroid is available only in the U.S.

Color	Dosage	Brands	Weight Range
orange	25	Synthroid/Levoxyl/ Levothroid	16–23 kg/30–50 lbs
white	50	Synthroid/Levoxyl Levothroid/Eltroxin	24–39 kg/51–87 lbs
violet	75	Synthroid	40–51 kg/88–112 lbs
purple	75	Levoxyl	SAME
gray	75	Levothroid	SAME
olive	88	Synthroid/Levoxyl	52–59 kg/113–131 lbs
mint green	88	Levothroid	SAME
yellow	100	Synthroid/Levoxyl	60–66 kg/132–146 lbs

rose	112	Levothroid/Eltroxin Synthroid/Levoxyl Levothroid	67–74 kg/147–163 lbs
brown	125	Synthroid/Levoxyl	75–86 kg/164–190 lbs
purple	125	Levothroid	SAME
dark blue	137	Levoxyl	82–91 kg/180–200 lbs
blue	137	Levothroid	SAME
light blue	150	Synthroid/Levoxyl Levothroid/Eltroxin	87–101 kg/191–225 lbs
lilac	175	Synthroid	SPECIAL CASES
turquoise	175	Levoxyl/Levothroid	SAME
pink	200	Synthroid/Levoxyl Levothroid/Eltroxin	SAME
green	300	Synthroid/Levoxyl Levothroid/Eltroxin	SAME

Sources: 1. "Solving the puzzle of hypothyroidism." Physician literature, supplied by Knoll Pharma Inc., 1995. 2. Levoxyl Prescribing Information, Daniels Pharmaceuticals, Inc., 1994. 3. Levothroid Prescribing Information, Forest Pharmaceuticals, Inc., 1995. 4. Eltroxin Prescribing Information, GlaxoWellcome, Inc. 1995.

3. If pharmacists tempt you with a cheaper generic brand that is just as good, remember that you can have a quality brand for very little money anyway, so why settle for cheap wine? The bottom line is that you get what you pay for.

4. Watch for signs of hyperthyroidism (see the Hyper-alphabet in chapter 2). These symptoms mean that you're on too high of a dosage of thyroid hormone.

5. Watch for signs of hypothyroidism (see the Hypo-alphabet in chapter 2). These are signs that you're on too low a dosage of thyroid hormone.

6. Get a thyroid function test once every three months for the first couple of years after you begin your pills; then graduate once every six months; then graduate to annual tests.

What's in This Stuff, Anyway?

Thyroid hormone pills contain a number of excipients (substances added to a medicine which allow it to be formed into a shape and consistency). These include diluents, lubricants, binders, and disintegrants. The pills may contain acacia, lactose, magnesium stearate, povidone, confectioners sugar (which has corn starch), and talc. The lactose used in thyroid hormone pills is minimal; there is approximately 100 times the amount of lactose in one-half cup of whole milk as in one tablet of Synthroid, for example. If you're highly lactose intolerant, you can take your thyroid hormone pill together with a lactase enzyme.

When to Take Your Thyroid Hormone Pill

It's best to take thyroid hormone medication on an empty stomach around the same time every day. When your stomach's empty, the hormone is absorbed into your system more efficiently. Taking the pill at the same time every day helps you to establish your own pill routine while creating a balance of the hormone in your system. One study found that patients on thyroid hormone specifically for TSH suppression were better off waiting one hour after taking their pill in the morning before having breakfast. It was suspected that milk products had something to do with improving the absorption of the medication. If you're taking multivitamin pills or iron supplements, such as ferrous sulfate, take your thyroid hormone pill at least two hours in advance. Iron appears to bind to thyroid hormone, making less of it available for absorption by your body.

It's a good idea to get a weekly pill organizer; the main problem with taking daily medication is combating absentmindedness. Most of us lead busy, hectic lives and perform routine tasks without realizing we're doing them. For example, how often have you turned the stove off and then wondered on your way to work whether you actually did it or just thought you did? The same thing happens with taking a pill every day. *Did I take the pill? I don't* remember *taking it!* This can be a frustrating experience because once you doubt whether you've taken your medication, psychosomatic symptoms take over and you actually can begin to *feel* hypothyroid even though you're not. A pill organizer will help you keep track. Generally, thyroid medication is designed to linger in your system a long time, so skipping a pill every so often won't make a difference. However, if you just *think* you forgot your pill, the psychological effect of "knowing you forgot" is powerful, and phantom hypothyroidism can set in. (This is similar to a woman "suddenly getting cramps" when she discovers she has her period!) For the record, here's how thyroid replacement really works.

The effect of the thyroid pill you take today isn't felt until five to ten days *after* you take it. (This doesn't mean, though, that because you missed a dose and feel fine that you don't need your thyroid medication.) You will begin to feel better in about four to six weeks after starting on thyroid hormone. Most patients will take six to nine months to feel really well again. Furthermore, even if you were to stop taking thyroid hormone altogether, it would still take at least a month for all of the hormone to be used up by the body. The bottom line is that if you think you've forgotten to take your thyroid medication but aren't sure, skip it. Just take the pill the next day and carry on. You don't need to double your dose the way one does with birth control pills. However, taking two thyroid pills the next day won't harm you in any way. In fact, endocrinologists say that it doesn't matter if, on occasion, you miss one, or take two accidentally. Just don't make a habit of it!

Thyroid Hormone Replacement and Other Drugs

Because we all either combine various medications from time to time or take other daily medications for different health conditions, it's important to be aware of how thyroid hormone replacement medication interacts with other prescription and nonprescription drugs.

When combined with oral anticoagulants (Coumadin, Warfarin, Heparin). An anticoagulant, or blood thinner, helps prevent blood clotting and is prescribed for a variety of heart conditions or during or after surgical procedures. When combined with thyroid hormone, the anticoagulant can become more potent, which could cause minor hemorrhaging. Your doctor may need to reduce the dosage of Coumadin, Heparin, or Warfarin. This occurs only when initiating thyroxine therapy, not when patients are taking it chronically. When an elderly patient is on these drugs, thyroid levels should be tested every six months.

When combined with estrogen or birth control pills. This combination can increase your bound T_4 (thyroxine) readings, as discussed in chapter 7. It's best to get your thyroid levels checked once a year if you're on the Pill or Premarin or are taking estrogen hormone for other reasons. "Free" T_4 remains the same, however.

When combined with insulin or oral hypoglycemics for diabetics. This combination lowers the effect of insulin, which means that your doctor may have to increase your insulin dosage. This occurs only when you begin to take thyroid hormone tablets. After both medications are adjusted, you should be fine. If you're diabetic, however, it's a good idea to get your thyroid levels checked once a year.

When combined with Dilantin. When combined with anticonvulsants, drugs such as Dilantin, are prescribed for epilepsy; it helps to prevent seizures. This combination lowers your bound T_4 levels. This doesn't mean that you'll become hypothyroid, but your thyroid tests will be more difficult to interpret.

When combined with laxatives (such as Metamucil), coffee, or alcohol. Thyroid hormone and anything that affects the digestive system should be taken as many hours apart as possible to ensure better absorption of the thyroid medication.

When combined with cholestyramine (Questran). This drug is prescribed for people who have high cholesterol levels. When combined with thyroid hormone, this drug lowers the absorption of thyroxine. Therefore, the two should not be taken together. A space of three to four hours between each is recommended, and thyroid hormone should be taken first.

When combined with antidepressants. If you're on thyroid hormone replacement and are taking any one of the following antidepressant drugs—Elavil, Ascendin, Etrafon, Limbitral, Pamelor, Surmontil, Tofranil, Tofranil P.M., Triavil, or Norpramin—the antidepressant drug will become more potent. This can also lead to abnormal heart rhythms. This only happens when you just begin your thyroid medication, however, and it tapers off when your medications are balanced. Make sure you get your thyroid levels checked every year, and inform whoever is managing your antidepressant medication that you are in fact taking thyroid hormone.

The Effects of Lithium

Lithium is prescribed for bipolar disorder (formerly known as manic depression). Even if your thyroid is functioning normally, lithium can cause hypothyroidism; 8 to 19% of people on lithium become hypothyroid. Lithium has also been known to cause goiter, hyperthyroidism, and to trigger Graves' disease. This can be a problem because the hypothyroidism can either cause depression or make your existing depression worse. This may result in an increased dosage of lithium, worsening the undiagnosed hypothyroidism. The best way to avoid this potential nightmare is to make sure you inform whoever is monitoring your lithium that your thyroid function should first be checked. Then, insist that your thyroid levels are checked every six months while you're on lithium. In between checkups, you might want to keep a log of your moods on a day-to-day basis. If you're feeling unusually depressed for long periods of time, get your thyroid levels checked just in case. Once you're on thyroid hormone, there is no more concern regarding lithium. It can only affect the production of thyroid hormone within the thyroid gland; it has no effect on how thyroid hormone acts in the rest of the body.

Effects of Amiodarone

This is a drug used to treat atrial fibrillation, a heart rhythm problem. This drug contains a lot of iodine, and it has been found to induce both hypo- and hyperthyroidism; but in North America, where we have sufficient iodine, hypothyroidism is more common. It has also been found to accelerate Hashimoto's disease, but it does not cause it in people who don't suffer from it initially. Amiodarone causes hyperthyroidism if you have a toxic multinodular goiter. If you're vulnerable to thyroid disease, and you're on this drug, request an antithyroid antibody test just in case. Since the drug is stored in body fat, it can induce a thyroid problem up to 12 months after it has been stopped.

Additional Things to Keep in Mind

- You may nurse your baby while on thyroid hormone (thyroxine).
- You must continue to take your thyroid hormone pill when you're pregnant.
- You can take your thyroid hormone pill before you go for blood work; it won't affect the results in any way.
- The Red Cross *will* accept you as a blood donor if you are taking thyroxine and are healthy. (Do check with your doctor before

you give blood, though.)

- Doctors may sometimes order treadmill heart testing before they start you on thyroid hormone. Don't worry about this; your doctor just wants to be sure you have no evidence of heart disease before he or she prescribes thyroid medication. Why? Because if you do have coronary heart disease, you'll be prescribed a lower dose of thyroxine at first.

A Word About Dyes

Many diagnostic tests use contrast dyes to take pictures of organs such as the brain, gall bladder, kidney, and spinal cord. Angiograms are particular culprits in this respect, which may complicate thyroid-related heart problems. These dyes often contain iodine, which can trigger hyper- or hypothyroidism in someone who has a borderline or already diagnosed thyroid condition. The test results can also mislead a doctor to diagnose a primary thyroid condition in a person with a healthy thyroid gland. Just keep this in mind and request a thyroid test *after* one of these tests to make sure the thyroid condition actually exists.

Medications to Stay Away from While You're Hyperthyroid

- Avoid taking cough/cold medicines with decongestants. These drugs can cause restlessness and stimulate your heart. Since your heart is already being overstimulated by your hyperthyroid condition, you don't want to tempt fate and risk any added stimulation. (However, mild exercise and sexual activity are fine!)
- Avoid other stimulants such as caffeine (found in coffee and chocolate), alcohol, or tobacco. Again, these stimulants increase your heart rate.
- Avoid anything with excess iodine. Some prescription and over-the-counter drugs contain iodine, such as certain asthma medications, vitamin pills, cough medicines, suntan lotions, and salt substitutes. Make sure you read the labels before you take any

other medications while you're hyperthyroid. You should also stay away from kelp (seaweed) and cut down on eating seafood while you're hyperthyroid. The iodine in these substances can make your hyperthyroidism worse by triggering the thyroid gland to make more thyroxine with the extra iodine.

- Don't take Haldol if you're hyperthyroid. Haldol is a drug prescribed for certain psychiatric disorders (it's an antipsychotic) and is also widely used to control alcohol withdrawal for recovering alcoholics. Hyperthyroid patients taking Haldol may develop extreme stiffness or rigidity which could lead to the inability to walk. Not a good idea!
- If you've been prescribed propanalol to control your heart rate, and are asthmatic, propanalol can trigger asthma attacks. Make sure you consult with your doctor or pharmacist about your asthma before you go on propanalol.

Antithyroid Medication

The only time you'll take antithyroid medication is if you're hyperthyroid. The most commonly used antithyroid drugs are propylthiouracil (PTU), prescribed daily at 300 to 400 milligrams and tapazole (aka methimazole), prescribed daily at 30 to 40 milligrams. These drugs prevent the thyroid gland from manufacturing thyroid hormone, which causes the symptoms of hyperthyroidism to subside. You'll probably begin to feel better within two weeks, feel a difference by six weeks, and feel completely well again in ten to fourteen weeks. You'll most likely be on antithyroid medication anywhere from six to twelve months. Your doctor will check at six months, nine months, and twelve months to see if you still need it. If your thyroid gland now functions normally, your family doctor will still check you periodically to be sure that your thyroid hormone level (T_4) remains within the normal range or just above normal range.

Unlike thyroid hormone, if you forget a dose of antithyroid medication, you must double it on the next dose. Propylthiouracil is only potent for eight hours, so unlike thyroid hormone replacement, if you miss a day, it matters. However, methimazole has a much longer half-life and needs to be taken only once a day.

Side Effects

Some people develop various reactions to antithyroid medications. The reactions include rashes, itching, hives, joint pains, and sore throat and fever (symptoms of a low white blood count, which the drug also causes), jaundice, and in extremely rare cases, liver failure (a rare complication common to many prescription drugs). If this happens, stop taking the drug and call your doctor right away. Although these reactions could occur for any number of reasons that may have nothing to do with antithyroid drugs, you don't want to risk an allergy. At this point your doctor will check your white blood cell count and make sure it's normal. Even if it is, your allergy symptoms still may be due to the antithyroid drugs and your doctor will reconsider the antithyroid medication. If your white blood cell count is decreased, your doctor will then discuss another form of treatment such as radioactive iodine therapy or surgery. As discussed in several previous chapters, radioactive iodine therapy or surgery will leave you with a nonfunctioning thyroid gland, which will cause you to be hypothyroid. To balance this, you'll be placed on thyroid hormone replacement.

Notes of Caution

- Mothers on tapazole or methimazole should not breast-feed because the drug can pass to the child through the milk. However, mothers on a small dose of propylthiouracil can still nurse because this drug does not pass into the milk unless the dosage is large.
- You cannot donate blood to the Red Cross if you're taking antithyroid medication.

What About Alternatives to Thyroid Hormone Pills?

While there are many health problems that can be beautifully treated with herbal preparations or alternative therapies, thyroid disease just isn't one of them. I am frequently asked about herbs or kelp. Nothing replaces the thyroid hormone more exactly than pharmaceutically-prepared thyroid hormone replacement. Not Kentucky Fried Thyroid from a mammal, not kelp, not drops, or other herbal concoctions. Unless you're taking thyroid hormone replacement in pill form, you run the risk of becoming hyperthyroid or hypothyroid.

That said, if you want to incorporate alternative therapies into your life while taking thyroid hormone replacement, fine. Be it therapeutic massage, Ayurveda, iridology, or the host of complementary therapies available, the alternative world is your oyster. Just don't *substitute* kelp or any concoction for thyroid hormone replacement.

How to Use a Pharmacist

Having a good pharmacist is as important as having a good doctor; your health is at risk if either one is incompetent. Since medication plays an integral role in not only a thyroid patient's life but everyone's, pharmacists and doctors are equally responsible for monitoring our medication.

However, since the pharmaceutical industry is heavily legislated and lobbied, understanding who's in control of our drugs gets confusing. Basically, pharmaceutical products work like any other distribution network. Obviously the manufacturer in this case is the drug company, but it is the pharmacist who is the distributor, the doctor who *retails* the product—selling it to *us*—while we, the patients, are the consumers, or end users of the product. A doctor's prescription is really just a purchase order for the pharmacist, since prescription drugs can't be distributed without one! What's odd about this distribution network, though, is that we pay the distributor for the product instead of the retailer, who actually sold us the product. So if the sale is made before we even get to the pharmacy, and the pharmacist doesn't actually sell us anything, what *is* the pharmacist's job?

It is up to the pharmacist to fill in the blanks, not just fill the prescription. The pharmacist makes sure the doctor has ordered the correct drug for the correct condition, and makes sure the patient understands how to take, store, and refill the medication in appropriate quantities. The pharmacist should also take medical histories and make sure patients aren't seeing more than one doctor for the same prescription or using conflicting medications. This happens a lot. For one thing, patients don't always tell their doctors about other physicians they're seeing, or doctors forget to update other physicians on patients they have in common.

Some Common Problems

A typical medication mess goes something like this: Mrs. Doe, a 70-year-old woman who has been on thyroid hormone replacement for years, runs out of thyroid hormone pills. She refills her prescription through the pharmacy that holds her original thyroid hormone prescription. A few days later, Mrs. Doe sees a new specialist for a health problem unrelated to her thyroid condition. The specialist routinely takes her medical history and inadvertently finds out that Mrs. Doe had her thyroid removed in the early 1960s to treat a goiter. Just to be thorough, the specialist asks her if she is taking thyroid hormone pills.

"Oh yes," she says, "but I've run out." Absentmindedly, Mrs. Doe forgot that she just refilled her thyroid hormone prescription two days ago, and in fact took a thyroid pill that morning! The specialist, being a good soul, asks Mrs. Doe what color her thyroid pills were (the color tells him what dosage she's on). "Blue," she replies. The specialist then writes her a prescription for a one-month supply of thyroid hormone at a strength of 150 micrograms (a blue pill).

"This will tide you over until you can get in to see your family doctor or endocrinologist for a new prescription," the specialist says. The specialist knows that sometimes patients can wait weeks for an appointment, and he doesn't want Mrs. Doe to become hypothyroid. When Mrs. Doe leaves the new specialist's office, she goes to a pharmacy across the street and hands over the prescription he gave her. "My new doctor gave me more medication," she says. Mrs. Doe doesn't have a clue what the prescription is for; she was preoccupied when the specialist gave it to her and doesn't realize it's just more thyroid hormone. The pharmacist fills the prescription.

"Make sure you take one pill every day until this bottle is empty, okay, Mrs. Doe?"

"Yes, thank you." Mrs. Doe heads home. The next morning she takes a thyroid pill from her new refilled supply and then takes a thyroid pill from her new one-month supply. She's now doubled her prescription without knowing it. By the time she finishes her one-month supply, she will be hyperthyroid from a thyroid hormone pill overdose.

So who's responsible for Mrs. Doe's overdose and inevitable hyperthyroidism? The specialist was trying to be thorough, the pharmacist made sure that Mrs. Doe understood how to take her medication, and Mrs. Doe was just following instructions. Despite this, the fault lies with both doctor and pharmacist alike. Obviously, Mrs. Doe was elderly and not entirely on the ball. The specialist should have first asked Mrs. Doe who she was seeing about her thyroid condition, and notified her "thyroid doctor" that she was out of pills. He then should have asked her which pharmacy she went to for her thyroid pills, and phoned the pharmacy to see if there was a refill on her prescription. At this point the pharmacy would have told the specialist that Mrs. Doe had in fact just refilled the prescription.

The problem also could have been caught by the new pharmacist. Here is the general line of questioning that would have prevented the problem:

Q: Are you taking any other medications?
A: Yes, but I don't remember what they're called.

Q: Did you get your other medications filled here?
A: No, they were filled at a pharmacy near my house.

Q: Where is your regular pharmacy located?
A: 22 Smith Street.

At this point, the new pharmacist should call Mrs. Doe's regular pharmacist and find out what other drugs she's taking to avoid any conflicts. When the Smith Street pharmacy tells this new pharmacist that Mrs. Doe is already on thyroid hormone replacement, the pharmacist should find out when she last had the thyroid medication dispensed, and then check back with the specialist who wrote the prescription to find out why additional thyroid pills were prescribed.

Here's another line of questioning that would have caught the problem:

Q: Did the doctor tell you what this medication is for?
A: I think so, but I've forgotten.

Q: This is thyroid medication. Are you taking any other thyroid medication? (An experienced pharmacist has seen this before in elderly patients.)
A: Yes, but I think my pills ran out.

Q: What pharmacy usually handles your thyroid medication?

Again, the pharmacist will check and find out what's really going on.

Other common problems revolve around pill quantities. For example, Ms. Brown, a 19-year-old woman, has just received a prescription for a six-month supply of thyroid hormone tablets with four repeats. She goes to the pharmacy and is asked by the pharmacist: "Do you want me to fill the whole prescription, or do you want to just come back for each repeat?"

"Which is cheaper?" she asks.

"Well, it'll cost you less for us to fill the whole thing now than it would to repeat the prescription," answers the pharmacist. (This is true, but doctors ask that medication be repeated for a reason.)

"Fill the whole thing!" she says. Problem: Instead of getting a six-month supply of pills, Ms. Brown is now getting a two-year supply. First, there is the shelf-life issue. Will the pills be as potent two years from now as they are when dispensed in six-month intervals? If they are less potent, Ms. Brown may wind up hypothyroid from stale thyroid pills. Second, will Ms. Brown assume that because she has enough medication for two years, she doesn't need to see her doctor for two years? A good pharmacist would have explained that the doctor ordered the pills in six-month intervals so that Ms. Brown could have her thyroid levels checked every six months and have her dosage adjusted if necessary.

Choosing a Pharmacist

As you can see from the discussion above, a good pharmacist must ask the right kind of questions to help prevent real health problems from happening, and be able to explain the medication thoroughly to the patient. But most of us use different criteria for choosing pharmacists than we use for choosing physicians. For example, we tend to want pharmacists who are in a convenient location and who provide prompt service. This is fine for a dry cleaner, but when we hire someone to distribute our medications to us, we need to be more selective. The following are some guidelines to use when choosing a pharmacist or assessing your current pharmacist.

1. How experienced is your pharmacist? Is his or her degree plainly displayed? If it isn't, find out if he or she is *really* qualified.
2. Does your pharmacist speak the same language as you? If you can't understand what your pharmacist says, switch!
3. How does your pharmacist treat other customers? Does he or she take the time to question them and carefully explain medications, or is the pharmacist impatient and rude? Observing how your pharmacist behaves with other people should tell you a lot!
4. Is your pharmacist helpful and always willing to answer *your* questions? Or does he or she shunt you aside and tell you to call your doctor?

By the same token, here are some guidelines for you to follow to make sure you're using your pharmacist correctly:

1. Do you have 12 different pharmacists for 12 different prescriptions? If you do, it's a mistake. Always "bank" at the same pharmacy. That way, your medication records are always up-to-date. Many pharmacies now offer a computerized medication record system so that all of your prescriptions are regularly updated and cross-referenced. Try to look for this service if you can.
2. Always ask when you should take your medications: on an empty or full stomach, in the morning or night, and so forth. The doctor usually indicates this on the label, but double-check!
3. Always discuss dosage requirements (one pill each day, one pill twice a day, and so on) and appropriate quantities (getting a one-month supply versus a one-year supply) with the pharmacist.
4. Always ask where to store your medication. Did you know that bathrooms are the *worst* place to store any medication? Moisture can get into the medication and affect the drug's potency, and children can easily access it in the bathroom.
5. Always ask the pharmacist how long a shelf life your medication has. Expiration dates vary depending on how long pharmacists have had the medication on *their* shelves. Most thyroid hormone pills don't have an expiration date *listed* on their labels.

Thyroid medication is crucial to patients who want to maintain normal thyroid levels, and balancing thyroid medication is the key to prolonged health. Since the medication is usually lifelong, you should work at establishing a rapport as well as a long-term relationship with your pharmacist, just as you would with your doctor. That way, as you age and may become more dependent on a variety of medications simultaneously, your pharmacist can act as another safety net in the health care system. Recent surveys show that half the people who take prescription medicine are not taking it correctly. This disturbing statistic reveals miscommunication at both the doctor-patient and pharmacist-patient levels. By becoming more responsible with your thyroid medication, and taking the time to use your pharmacist correctly, you can help prevent potential medication messes while maintaining your health. The next chapter will discuss other maintenance tips for staying healthy, as well as new thyroid research on the horizon that will help make the upkeep of normal thyroid levels less stressful for patients, doctors, and pharmacists.

I'm Cured—Now What?

It's one thing to be diagnosed and treated for your thyroid condition; it's quite another to maintain good health and a balance of thyroid hormone in your body. There are several hurdles that thyroid patients need to leap when it comes to staying healthy. The first one is medication, discussed in the last chapter. The second one is aging. Thyroid hormone requirements change as we get older; we usually require less hormone as the years go by. Keeping on top of your medication, seeing your doctor for regular checkups, and monitoring your dosage are all crucial. The third hurdle is nutrition. Although good nutrition is essential for *everyone's* good health, thyroid patients are more sensitive to poor nutrition because it can aggravate their conditions.

The Thyroid Outpatient

There comes a point in your thyroid odyssey where you are in fact "cured," even though you may be on thyroid medication for the rest of your life. Essentially, you'll go from being a thyroid patient to a thyroid *out*patient. Instead of checking in with your doctor every few weeks as you receive various treatments and therapies for your thyroid condition, your thyroid disorder will have been successfully treated at this point, and your thyroid hormone levels will now be balanced through thyroid hormone replacement. You'll only need to see your doctor either every six months or annually to get your thyroid levels checked and have your medication dosage monitored. This routine generally doesn't change unless you develop a health problem that complicates your existing thyroid disorder or medication, or you experience difficulty in balancing your thyroid medication. Basically, you'll graduate from patient to outpatient as you get healthier.

What If I Refuse Treatment?

Most people with a thyroid disorder will simply get worse without treatment. In fact, one hundred years ago, hyperthyroidism and hypothyroidism were fatal diseases because they led to cardiovascular failure. In the first case, the heart is overworked; while in the second case, the heart muscles go limp and flabby, causing heart failure as well.

As discussed in chapter 4, some cases of thyroiditis will resolve without treatment. In many cases, hyperthyroidism due to Graves' disease burns out after about 15 years, but you would be a physical wreck by then without treatment. And, very occasionally, mild hyperthyroidism due to Graves' disease has gone into spontaneous remission without treatment.

The issue of refusing treatment is gaining popularity with a variety of chronic conditions for which there is no cure. For example, in many cases of infertility, people decide not to pursue treatment because their condition isn't life threatening; it simply means they cannot have biological children. In many cases of terminal cancer or other terminal illness, many people decide that treatment to prolong their lives by a few months isn't worth sacrificing the *quality* of life. Since thyroid disease can almost always be successfully treated, there doesn't seem to be a logical reason to refuse treatment.

Finally, more than a few thyroid patients refuse conventional treatment because they believe they are suffering from a syndrome called Wilson's syndrome. This is a nonexistent condition that was coined by Dr. Wilson in Orlando, Florida. There is no scientific basis for his syndrome, wherein he claims that patients have slow metabolism due to poor T_3 conversion. In this case, he recommends treatment with T_3 instead of T_4. Anyone diagnosed with Wilson's syndrome should seek treatment with an endocrinologist.

Aging

If you developed a thyroid disorder in your late teens or early twenties, don't be surprised if your dosage is altered as you approach 30. Stress levels increase as you take on more career and family responsibilities, and women planning pregnancy will need to be monitored more closely. If your thyroid disorder develops in your thirties, it's likely that either stress or pregnancy has triggered the disorder initially, or you may need to adjust your dosage as a result of certain stresses or pregnancy. Then, as you head into your forties, you may find that your dosage needs adjusting; some of us settle into a more secure lifestyle by this time or find our lives are beginning anew as a result of career or lifestyle changes (divorce, second marriages, and so on).

When thyroid disorders develop in your forties, dosages may need to be frequently adjusted as you approach 50. Women entering menopause will need to keep a close watch on their levels, osteoporosis can be a concern, and other age-related health problems can develop or catch up with you that can affect thyroid hormone levels. For example, smoking, poor diet, and lack of exercise can affect your overall health in terms of heart rate, cholesterol levels, and so forth. All of this might affect your thyroid hormone dosage. When thyroid disorders occur in your 50s and early 60s, your health picture will most likely be fully developed by now. In other words, other problems will have already unfolded, such as high blood pressure, osteoporosis, high cholesterol, and angina. At this point your thyroid hormone levels will be set according to other medications you're on or other health conditions that have manifested over the years. If you're a woman, you'll most likely be through menopause, and your estrogen levels will be balanced by this point, too.

Thyroid After 65

Many people first develop thyroid problems after 65. Several studies show that thyroid illness is very much a disease of the elderly that often goes undiagnosed. Hypothyroidism is twice as common as hyperthyroidism in people over 65. One study indicates that as many as 4% of the over-65 population have undiagnosed hypothyroidism, while 2% have undiagnosed hyperthyroidism. Subclinical hypothyroidism (see chapter 2) affects 5% of the general population and roughly 15% of all women over 60. Left untreated, subclinical hypothyroidism will turn into blatant hypothyroidism at the rate of 5 to 20% per year, but the symptoms will be masked or exacerbated by aging. Chances are, if you're in this age group and have just developed a thyroid problem, you're a woman; women tend to live longer than men. However, it's difficult for doctors to diagnose thyroid disorders in women after 65 because they may not be able to feel the thyroid gland on an older woman's body. By the time women reach this age, the thyroid falls down into the chest and is hidden behind the breastbone. In fact, when a doctor can actually feel the thyroid gland of an older women, it's probably not healthy and is really a goiter. So to combat this problem, the TSH levels of most women over 50 (and certainly after 65) are routinely screened. If you do develop a thyroid disorder after 65, you'll be treated like anyone else depending on your condition, and you'll be put on thyroid hormone replacement. Generally, your dosage may be adjusted every few years to prevent overdosing on thyroid hormone.

Nutrition

Thyroid hormone helps distribute ingested food appropriately throughout your body. When the thyroid gland becomes either overactive or underactive, there are a number of nutritional concerns to address, and dietary changes you can make to help your body adjust to the problem. However, once you're treated and your levels are balanced, you'll need once again to readjust your eating habits to meet the needs of normal thyroid levels, and continue to eat well to give your replacement hormone tablet the help it needs to do its job.

Calories

The average adult with a healthy thyroid gland requires about 1,680 calories a day to maintain the right energy balance and ideal weight. When you're hyperthyroid, you need to increase your daily calories by 160 to 200% just to maintain the same energy and weight. With hyperthyroidism, protein and fats are not broken down normally; there is a decrease in fat stores and a lowering of the triglyceride and cholesterol levels. That means you'll be eating a lot more than you usually do to compensate for this energy loss. But the honeymoon does end. (Sometimes, however, you might gain a little weight because you become less active when you're hyperthyroid due to a very real exhaustion that sets in.) When you're "cured" and your thyroid levels are back to normal, you'll need to cut down on your calories or you'll definitely gain weight.

When you're hypothyroid, you need only about half the calories of an average adult to maintain your energy and weight. Here, there is an increase in fat stores, while your triglyceride and cholesterol levels rise. This could lead to heart trouble if you don't cut down on fat. In fact, unless you cut down on your overall calorie intake by 50 to 60%, you'll gain weight by eating what you normally do. Once your thyroid levels are balanced again, you'll be able to increase your calorie intake to what it was before you became hypothyroid.

Since your thyroid levels may fluctuate from time to time as you age or develop other health conditions, you'll have to get used to fluctuating your eating habits to keep up.

Food for Hyperthyroidism

Thyroid hormone affects your entire digestive system from mouth to bowels. Your thyroid has a hand in food absorption, gastric emptying, secretion of digestive juices, and motility of the digestive tract. When you're hyperthyroid, despite a voracious appetite, you might lose weight, have diarrhea, develop mild anemia, and suffer bone loss as calcium is taken out of the blood and excreted in the urine. The calcium loss could lead to osteoporosis in women. Generally, premenopausal women need 1,000 milligrams of calcium a day, while a postmenopausal woman needs 1,200 to 1,500 milligrams of calcium daily. But you can help ease the unpleasantness by controlling what you eat. Increase your calcium intake by consuming more butter, cream, cheese, and other dairy products. This will also help keep your weight up. Peanut butter, mayonnaise, and animal fat help as well. To reduce diarrhea, cut down on fruit juices and fresh fruits. Peanut butter is also good for binding. Hyperthyroid people sometimes develop sudden lactose intolerance. This can lead to gas and other unpleasantries. Cut out the milk products in this case and take a calcium supplement, and get your fat from the other foods mentioned above.

Stay away from caffeine, alcohol, and nicotine, which may stimulate your heart. You may want to take vitamin supplements as well. (Vitamins A, D, and E are stored in body fat and could get excreted if you're hyperthyroid.) When you're balanced again, you'll need to cut down on your fat and calcium intake.

Food for Hypothyroidism

Hypothyroidism causes poor appetite (despite weight gain), constipation, *pronounced anemia,* and a yellowing of the skin due to poor distribution of carotene, or vitamin A. You'll need lots of fiber: bran, whole grain breads, beans, nuts, seeds, fruits, and vegetables. This will help keep your bowels moving regularly, since you'll most likely be constipated. To lower cholesterol and triglycerides, reduce your intake of foods with high cholesterol: organ meats, eggs, shrimp, animal fats, and dairy products. Instead, substitute vegetable fats such as corn oil or some margarines. Drink a lot of fluids to excrete the buildup of various vitamins and minerals in your system, and start an exercise routine. Nutritionists recommend walking about 15 minutes a day at least 3 times a week over a long-term basis. After your thyroid levels are balanced, you can eat normally, but it's a good idea to keep up your hypothyroid "routine" as well. Why stop exercising? It's good for you anyway. Why stop eating fiber?

Nutrition for "Euthyroidism"

Euthyroid, as mentioned several times throughout the book, is the term used to describe normal thyroid levels. Basically, the healthiest diet is combining a hyperthyroid and hypothyroid diet and routine. In other words, eat a lot of calcium foods as well as high-fiber foods; try to use vegetable fats when you can and eat plenty of fruit, but continue to cut down on caffeine and alcohol. And remember to exercise. Use your common sense to benefit from both thyroid worlds. When your thyroid levels are back to normal and your treatments are complete, make an appointment with a nutritionist. All hospitals have nutritionists on staff, or ask your family doctor to refer you to one. Put together a realistic food plan with the nutritionist that meets your dietary and lifestyle needs.

Eating healthy will help your synthetic hormone pill work better because your digestion will be better able to absorb the hormone. If you happen to be someone who was *successfully* treated for hyperthyroidism on antithyroid medication and are not on thyroid hormone replacement at all, try to stay away from foods rich in iodine, which may retrigger your hyperthyroidism: iodized salt, seafood, kelp, and various medications or vitamin supplements listed in the previous chapter. Check with your nutritionist to create a sensible diet.

Cutting Dietary Fat

It's only natural that you want to eat well and be as healthy as you can possibly be today. For most of us, that means making some changes to our diet. Women who eat low fat diets and exercise have much lower rates of heart disease and stroke.

Eating well essentially means eating less fat, more fruits, all colors of vegetables, and lots of whole grains for fiber.

Good Fats/Bad Fats

Dietary fat is by far the most damaging element in the Western diet. This includes meats, dairy products, and vegetable oils. Other sources of fat include coconuts (60% fat), peanuts (78% fat), and avocados (82% fat). The latest theory is that diets with only 20% of calories from fat will probably serve you well. Though it's hard to know the difference between good fats and bad fats. There *is* a difference.

Olive oil, for example, is a good fat. It's a monounsaturated fat that tends to decrease the low density lipids (LDLs) in your bloodstream. LDL is also known as "bad" cholesterol. When LDL is decreased, the good cholesterol, high density lipids (HDLs) are increased.

Omega-3 oils, which are found mainly in fatty fish, have been proven beneficial to the heart and may also be associated with a protection against tumors. Fish containing these oils are salmon (natural only, not farm-raised), mackerel, sable, whitefish, herring, and sardines. Apparently, in order to derive any protection, you must eat these fishes frequently.

High-quality sesame oil or corn oil are also considered better oils to cook with. Sesame oil is also found in Japanese diets.

Solid evidence

The best way to determine bad fat is to see how solid it remains at room temperature. Things like lard, butter, margarine, and solid vegetable shortening, for example, are very bad fats. They're high in saturated fat and should be avoided. In fact, the way the fat looks prior to ingesting it is the way it will look when it lines your arteries. So, if you're lured into the low-calorie world of margarine and solid vegetable shortening, don't be fooled: they're no better than plain butter or lard because they contain *trans-fatty acids,* which have been linked to cardiovascular disease. Trans-fatty acids are made from the process of hydrogenation (this is what solidifies various oils).

Saturated fat

Here's the definition of saturated fats: anything that stimulates your body to make cholesterol. This is like giving yourself a cholesterol stimulant and is *worse* than foods naturally high in cholesterol. Foods high in saturated fats include chocolate, tropical oils (which is why coconut oil-popped popcorn is bad news), and liquid oils other than olive or canola (aka rapeseed) oils. Even though olive and canola oils still contain saturated fats, they have a higher smoking temperature than other liquid oils, which helps reduce the fat.

Modern milk

We consume a lot of milk in North America. In the United States, each person consumes roughly 350 pounds of milk per year, which is equal to roughly 72 gallons of milk. That translates into one cow for every second person. However, because of the heating procedures, homogenization, sterilization, addition of other ingredients such as vitamin D, hormones, antibodies, and other chemicals in milk, many people question whether it's still "nature's perfect food." When you consider that 75% of all dairy cows are artificially inseminated, milk somehow loses its wholesome persona.

The interesting thing about modern milk is that before we were able to store and preserve milk, most of the dairy products consumed were limited to fermented dairy foods, such as yogurt and kefir, which contain enzymes and bacteria that help to digest dairy.

Animal milk (goat, sheep, or donkey) was once reserved for mothers who couldn't breast-feed, but the huge quantities of animal milk humans ingest today were never intended by nature.

It's probably not entirely practical to stop consuming all dairy products, so here's the low-down on milk products:
- whole milk is made up of 48% calories from fat
- 2% milk gets 37% of its calories from fat
- 1% milk gets 26% of its calories from fat
- skim milk is completely fat-free
- cheese gets 50% of its calories from fat, unless its skim milk cheese
- butter gets 95% of its calories from fat
- yogurt gets 15% of its calories from fat

Trimming the Fat

The best way to cut your dietary fat is to simply read labels. A product that boasts fewer calories can mean anything from low sodium to low sugar, but not necessarily fewer fat grams. Labels that boast "lower in fat" need to be compared to something. For example, anything may be lower than lard or butter. If you read a label that boasts "no cholesterol, this probably means no animal fats, but could contain saturated fats, such as vegetable oil, which will raise your cholesterol levels anyway! Other label tricks include lowering the serving size. For instance, I actually fell for a label that screamed only 89 calories in big fat letters on potato crispy somethings. After I consumed a good portion of the box, I realized it was 89 calories per suggested serving, or *six* potato crisps (which, incidentally, weren't even made from real potatoes).

Some of the most fattening products are sold as health foods: granola bars (200 calories with roughly 50% derived from fat), carob and yogurt candies, and even low fat frozen yogurt can be high in fat, especially, if your frozen yogurt is topped with fattening goodies.

Good fat isn't as hard to find as you think. Any of these are considered good fats: whole grains, beans, nuts, and seeds, and the good oils mentioned above.

What you probably know . . . but may not

I hate to sound like your mother, but please remember that broiling, baking, steaming, poaching, roasting, or microwaving foods are healthier than frying or deep-frying. Vegetables are good steamed and now even boiled! Apparently, boiled vegetables are now thought to contain a thermoresistant substance that may have a protective effect against certain cancers. Steaming and roasting vegetables are fine, too. Here are some more fat-fighting tips.

- Whenever you refrigerate animal fat (as in soups, stews, or curry dishes), skim the fat from the top before reheating and serving.
- To cut some fat out of canned goods (soups, tuna, etc.), pour the contents through a coffee filter first.

- Substitute something else for butter: yogurt (great on potatoes), low-fat cottage cheese, or jams and jellies. For sandwiches, any condiment without butter, margarine, or mayonnaise is fine, i.e., mustard, yogurt, etc.
- Powdered nonfat milk is high in calcium and low in fat. Substitute it for any recipe calling for milk or cream.
- Dig out fruit recipes for dessert. Things like sorbet with low-fat yogurt topping can still be elegant.
- Season low-fat foods well. That way you won't miss the flavor fat adds.
- Good carbohydrates are products with polysaccharide glucose (cereal grains, veggies, beans); bad carbohydrates are monosaccharide or disaccharide sugars (fruit, honey, dairy foods, refined sugar, other sweeteners).
- Good protein comes from vegetable sources (whole grains and bean products); bad proteins come from animal sources.

Finally, many North Americans are substituting low-fat turkey meat for red meat. It's a good start. If you have to have beef, keep in mind that it varies in fat content. "Prime" beef carries the highest fat content; "choice" has less, while "select" has the least. Lean beef is apparently an oxymoron, since beef isn't bred to be lean.

Research on the Horizon

The last census of the World Health Organization on global health problems indicated that more than 200 million people in the world suffered from thyroid disease in one form or another. In iodine-deficient countries, 1.5 billion people (28.9% of the world's population) are at risk for thyroid disease. There is a great deal of research going into the causes, diagnosis, and treatment of thyroid disease. However, different parts of the world are involved in different thyroid research.

The Underdeveloped World

In underdeveloped countries, goiters, cretinism, and retardation are still widespread. Currently, researchers are trying to find out what other substances besides iodine in food and water can trigger thyroid disease. Research funds are also being used to bring standard North American newborn screening methods to other parts of the world. Ironically, poor nutrition is by far the most common cause of thyroid disease worldwide. Fighting iodine deficiency is still a problem, but public health organizations are trying to distribute iodized food and iodine supplements. However, fighting famine is a far more prevalent concern right now. It's hard enough to deliver enough wheat and flour; iodized salt is even more difficult.

However, certain foods in the underdeveloped world seem to interfere with iodine absorption, causing either goiters or cretinism. In Africa, for example, cassava is a major diet component. Even when iodine quantities are sufficient, people who have diets rich in cassava can suffer from iodine deficiency or iodine overdose. The same thing is happening with well water in parts of South America. This is currently being researched.

As discussed in chapter 1, the World Health Organization (WHO) and UNICEF, with the technical support of ICCIDD are trying to implement massive Universal Salt Iodization (USI) programs. Food stuffs such as bread, oil, and water can all be iodized very easily. Iodizing cows milk and animal feed are other options being explored, as well. Mineral water is another way of correcting iodine deficiency. Studies show that because of its low sodium concentrations, it's a good solution to iodine deficiency in low sodium diets.

The Developed World

Thyroid research in developed countries is far more sophisticated. There is considerable research on the effects of all kinds of radiation on the thyroid gland, as well as refining radioactive iodine therapy. For example, in the future it may be possible to cure hyperthyroidism without causing hypothyroidism. This has to do with calculating more precise dosages of radioactive iodine, and pinpointing finite regions of the thyroid gland.

The most intensive area of thyroid research is being conducted on the nature of autoimmune disease, autoimmune thyroid disease, and the accompanying eye complications. If thyroid researchers can find out what triggers autoimmune diseases, it's possible that a vaccine to prevent autoimmune thyroid diseases can be developed.

Other research projects involve the investigation of thyroid hormones and how they interact with crucial body functions and development. For example, the effect of thyroid hormone on brain development, the central nervous system, gene regulation, and the gastrointestinal tract are all projects in the works.

Funding

Although thyroid "technology" has certainly come a long way, only a fraction of medical research funds are allocated to thyroid research. Considering the fact that we are currently amidst epidemics such as AIDS and certain kinds of cancer, treatable conditions such as thyroid disorders are not top priorities at the moment.

In women's health issues, breast cancer, ovarian cancer, and AIDS are the main medical crises. It's far more important to allocate funding to these diseases than to thyroid disease at this point. It should be noted, though, that postpartum thyroid disease is making considerable headway on the thyroid research front, and as female baby boomers age, you can bet that thyroid disease and menopause will become a major research project.

1995: Year of the Thyroid

The year 1995 was especially hyperactive for thyroid awareness. January was declared National Thyroid Awareness Month in the United States (June is Thyroid Awareness Month in Canada). In September 1995, a historic meeting took place in the world of thyroid. It was the formation of an international consortium of thyroid organizations from around the world, called Thyroid Federation International (TFI). As one of the founding members of TFI, it was an extremely gratifying experience to see so many thyroid organizations come together.

TFI organizations, listed in the resource section, have a common mission:

- to educate and give moral support to thyroid patients around the world;
- to promote awareness of thyroid disorders;
- to work with thyroid specialists to update general physicians and other health professionals to improve recognition of, testing, and treatment of thyroid disorders;
- to encourage physicians and other health professionals to consider thyroid disease as a subspecialty; and
- to raise funds to support thyroid research.

Right now, TFI is interested in working with ICCIDD, WHO, and UNICEF to help eliminate iodine deficiency worldwide. It's also interested in developing guidelines regarding nuclear reactor accidents and potassium iodide (see chapter 11). Other areas TFI hopes to improve are neonatal screening for congenital hypothyroidism; screening women after childbirth, of whom 5 to 18% will develop a thyroid condition (see chapters 4 and 7); screening for subclinical hypothyroidism (see chapter 2 and above); and educating the public on sources of excessive iodine, such as kelp, dulse, and seaweed, which can trigger a thyroid problem. As I mentioned in chapter 12, taking these substances as an alternative to medical treatment isn't a good idea.

Thyroid and Our Furry Friends

Before I sign off, I thought you should know that pets are not immune to thyroid disorders any more than they are to heart problems, cancers, and all the other human ailments.

Hyperthyroidism is rarely seen in dogs, but tends to occur more often in cats. These cats will have a good appetite, accompanied by weight loss, agitation, and nervousness. When examined, hyperthyroid cats have very fast heart rates as well. Benign thyroid tumors are also common in cats.

Hypothyroidism, rarely seen in cats, seems to affect certain breeds of dogs, such as golden retrievers, Doberman pinschers, dachshunds, Irish setters, miniature schnauzers, Great Danes, poodles, boxers, and beagles. Look for obesity, lethargy, greasy thick skin, droopy face, heat seeking, and hair loss on the trunk. Thyroid-related heart disease with an enlarged heart and rhythm disorders occurs in Great Danes, Dobermans, and boxers. Finally, budgies, believe it or not, are prone to iodine deficiency and goiters!

Treatment for hyperthyroid dogs involves thyroid hormone replacement (they need 10 to 20 times the dose as we humans). Hypothyroid cats will be given antithyroid medication. Surgery on the hyperthyroid cat is a risk due to the fast heart rate. As for budgies—treatment varies on cost-effectiveness. Talk to your veterinarian for more information.

As research and technology continue to move forward, in the meantime you should know your thyroid history and make sure you communicate your thyroid legacy to your children. That way, potential thyroid patients will know who they are and be conscious of obvious thyroid disease symptoms as they age, and their doctors will be alerted to the possibility of a thyroid disorder in the future.

You can also become active in a thyroid foundation that helps to raise money for thyroid research. This is a good way to work out your thyroid frustration. You can also start your own local thyroid foundation chapter, or form a local thyroid association or support group. I know of at least four organizations which began this way since the first edition of this book. In fact, funding for research and education usually starts at the patient level. For example, the basis for AIDS research and education started in the basements, bedrooms, and living rooms of angry, committed people who wanted something done about the epidemic, while the first thyroid foundation was started by an elderly woman with Graves' disease who was frustrated with the lack of educational material available for patients. And I wrote this book because nobody else *had*.

The best thing you can do to help educate the public on thyroid disease is to pass on what you know to other thyroid patients and doctors. Recommend books, articles, or pamphlets you come across on thyroid disease. And don't be afraid to ask questions or start conversations with "I read that. . . ." Good luck and good health.

Appendix

Where to Go for More Information

Note: Because of the volatile nature of many health and non-profit organizations, some of the addresses and phone numbers below may have changed since this list was compiled. Many of these organizations will have e-mail addresses, which may not have been available at the time of this writing. E-mail addresses will be included in future editions of this book as more organizations go online. Increasingly, though, lists like this one at the back of a book are going the way of the dinosaur. Many resources can be found through the Internet (see Thyroid Online at the end of this list).

General

Thyroid Foundation of America, Inc.
Ruth Sleeper Hall 350
Massachussetts General Hospital
Boston, MA 02114
(617) 726-8500
1-800-832-8321
Fax (617) 726-4136
Maryland Chapter (301) 775-7553
Tri-State Chapter (212) 241-1501

Thyroid Foundation of Canada
1040 Gardiners Road, Suite C
Kingston, Ontario K7P 1R7
Phone/Fax (613) 634-3426
1-800-267-8822
Web site: http://www.io.org/~thyroid/Canada.html
e-mail address: thyroid@limestone.kosone.com
e-mail re: website: thyroid@io.org

The Thyroid Foundation of Texas
P.O. Box 820195
Houston, TX 77282-0195
(713) 496-4460
Fax (713) 496-6465

Thyroid Society for Education & Research
7515 S. Main Street, Suite 545
Houston, TX 77030
(713) 799-9909
1-800-THYROID
Fax (713) 779-9919

Autoimmune Disorders
American Autoimmune Related Diseases Association, Inc.
Michigan National Bank Bldg.
14475 Gratiot Avenue
Detroit, MI 48205
(313) 371-8600
Fax (313) 372-1512

National Association for Rare Disorders (NORD)
P.O. Box 8923
New Fairfield, CT 06812-1783
1-800-999-NORD

Childhood Thyroid Cancer in Belarus, Ukraine, and Russia
Children of Chernobyl Canadian Fund
1555 Bloor Street West
Toronto, Ontario
(416) 532-2223

Congenital Hypothyroidism
CHAPS (Congenital Hypothyroidism and Parents Support Group)
8 Rockhill Court
Edwardsville, IL 62025
(618) 692-1761

Graves' Disease
National Graves' Disease Foundation
2 Tsitsi Court
Brevard, NC 28712
(704) 877-5251 or send SASE with your information request

Nederlandse Vereniging van Graves Patenten
Heemskerk Klein Elsbroek 3
2182 TE Hillegom
Holland

Hair Loss

American Hair Loss Council
1-800-274-8717

Buyer's Guide to Wigs and Hairpieces: Write Ruth L. Weintraub,
420 Madison Avenue, Suite 406
New York, NY 10017
(212) 838-1333

Edith Imre Foundation for Loss of Hair
30 West 57th Street
New York, NY 10019
(212) 757-8160
Wig Hotline (212) 765-8397

Iodine Deficiency Disorders (IDD)

International Council for Control of Iodine Deficiency Disorders (ICCIDD)
J.T. Dunn, M.D.
Box 511, University of Virginia Medical Center
Charlottesvile, VA 22908

Nuclear Medicine

Society of Nuclear Medicine
475 Park Avenue South
New York, NY 10016
(212) 889-0717

Thyroid Eye Disease

T.E.D. (Thyroid Eye Disease)
Lea House
21 Troarn Way
Chudleigh, Devon TQ13 OPP
England

Thyroid Specialists

American Thyroid Association, Inc.
Montefiore Medical Center
111 East 210th Street
Bronx, NY 10467
(718) 882-6047
Fax (718) 882-6085
Physician referral: 1-800-542-6687

The Endocrine Society
4350 East West Highway, Suite 500
Bethesda, MD 20814-4410
(301) 941-0200
Fax (301) 941-0259

American Association of Clinical Endocrinologists
2589 Park Street
Jacksonville, FL 32204-4554
(904) 384-9490
Fax (904) 384-8124

Directories
American Medical Association
Division of Survey and Data Resources
515 North State Street
Chicago, IL 60610

The American Board of Medical Specialties
1 Rotary Center
Evanston, IL 60201

Marquis Who's Who
Macmillian Directory Division
3002 Glenview Road
Wilmette, IL 60091

International Thyroid Organizations

Associazione Italiana Basedowiani e Tiroidei
Borgo Felino 3
43100 Parma, Italy

British Thyroid Foundation
P.Ol Box HP22
Leeds, England
LS6 3RT

Thyroid Foundation of Australia
39 Waterside Crescent
Carramar NSW 2163
Australia

Schilddrusen Liga
Peter-Sander Strasse 15
D55252 Mainz-Kastel
Germany

Schildklierstichting Nederland
Postbus 138 1620 AC Hoorn
Netherlands

Thyroid Federation International

Associazione Italiana Basedowiani e Tiroidei (Italy)
British Thyroid Foundation (England)
CHAPS (Congenital Hypothyroidism and Parents Support) (U.S.A.)
National Graves' Disease Foundation (U.S.A.)
Nederlandse Vereniging van Graves Patenten (Netherlands)
Schilddrusen Liga (Germany)
Schildklierstichting Nederland (Netherlands)
T.E.D. (Thyroid Eye Disease) (England)
Thyroid Foundation of America, Inc. (U.S.A.)
Thyroid Foundation of Australia (Australia)
Thyroid Foundation of Canada (Canada)

Thyroid Online

Through the Internet, you may be able to participate in newsgroups and bulletin boards (public forums) on thyroid disease. These can be accessed through
either independent internet providers or through an interactive computer service, such as CompuServe, Prodigy, or America Online (AOL).

Literature searches are great ways of getting specific information. Medline is the best search service for medical journal articles (many of which are extremely technical), while it also has a separate search service called Cancerlit if you need information on thyroid cancer. CompuServe, Prodigy, or America Online all give you access to Medline. Medline is also available through many public and university libraries all over North America.

Another way of accessing good information is through a web browser, such as Netscape. By web browsing, you can go to various sites in cyberspace to find your information. When you don't know the worldwide web (www) address, you can use a search engine, such as Yahoo or Webcrawler, to search for what you want by simply typing in your topic. A search engine is essentially an index to the Internet. The more specific you can be in your search, the better. For example, if you want information on thyroid eye disease, don't type "thyroid disease" but "thyroid eye disease" or "Graves' disease."

Once the search engine completes its search, a list of various sites will appear, ranging from promotional websites, to pharmaceutical companies, to university bulletin boards, to pepperings of articles. When you go to a site, you can save or print the information. Flashing text (called hypertext) is a sign that you'll get more information when you click on it. This may even link you to other sites on the Internet.

To Get You Started

http://www.io.org/~thyroid/Canada.html
http://www.nef.carleton.ca/freeport/health/thyroid/menu

Bibliography

Resources for First Edition

Chapter 1

H. Jack Baskin, M.D., *How Your Thyroid Works, 3rd ed.* (1991, Adams Press, Chicago).

R. I. S. Bayliss and W. M. G. Tunbridge, *Thyroid Disease: The Facts* (1991, Oxford University Press, New York).

Joel I. Hamburger, M.D., F.A.C.P., *The Thyroid Gland: A Book for Thyroid Patients, 7th ed.* (1991, Joel Hamburger, M.D., Southfield, Michigan).

"The Thyroid Gland: A General Introduction," National Headquarters, Thyroid Foundation of Canada, Kingston, Ontario, Health Guide Series.

Lawrence C. Wood, M.D., F.A.C.P., David S. Cooper, M.D., F.A.C.P., and Chester Ridgway, M.D., F.A.C.P., *Your Thyroid: A Home Reference* (1990, Ballantine Books, New York).

Chapter 2

J. Malcolm O. Arnold, "The Heart and the Thyroid Gland" (Summary of a talk presented to Thyroid Foundation of Canada, January 27, 1987).

H. Jack Baskin, M.D., *How Your Thyroid Works, 3rd ed.* (1991, Adams Press, Chicago).

R. I. S. Bayliss and W. M. G. Tunbridge, *Thyroid Disease: The Facts* (1991, Oxford University Press, New York).

Daniel Drucker, M.D., interviewed, 1991.

Leslie M. C. Goldenberg, M.D., F.R.C.P., interviewed, 1991.

Joel I. Hamburger, M.D., F.A.C.P., *The Thyroid Gland: A Book for Thyroid Patients, 7th ed.* (1991, Joel Hamburger, M.D., Southfield, Michigan).

Russell Joffe, M.D., "The Thyroid and Psychiatric Illness" (Lecture presented to Thyroid Foundation of Canada, November 30, 1991).

William G. Paterson, M.D., "The Gastrointestinal Tract and Thyroid Disease" (*Thyrobulletin*, Summer 1992).

"To Confirm the Clinical Diagnosis," "Hypothyroidism," "Graves' Disease," National Headquarters, Thyroid Foundation of Canada, Kingston, Ontario, Health Guide Series.

Robert Volpé, M.D., interviewed, 1991.

Lawrence C. Wood, M.D., F.A.C.P., David S. Cooper, M.D., F.A.C.P., and E. Chester Ridgway, M.D., F.A.C.P., *Your Thyroid: A Home Reference* (1990, Ballantine Books, New York).

Chapter 3

H. Jack Baskin, M.D., *How Your Thyroid Works, 3rd ed.* (1991, Adams Press, Chicago).

R. I. S. Bayliss and W. M. G. Tunbridge, *Thyroid Disease: The Facts* (1991, Oxford University Press, New York).

Dr. Leslie J. DeGroot, Professor of Medicine, Head of Thyroid Research, University of Chicago, "Graves' Disease" (*Thyrobulletin*, Autumn 1990).

Joel I. Hamburger, M.D., F.A.C.P., *The Thyroid Gland: A Book for Thyroid Patients, 7th ed.* (1991, Joel Hamburger, M.D., Southfield, Michigan).

Dr. Jeffrey J. Hurwitz, Lecture, June 12, 1982, Topic: Thyroid Related Eye Diseases (Summary of Remarks, Thyroid Foundation of Canada).

"Graves' Disease," "Graves' Eye Disease," National Headquarters, Thyroid Foundation of Canada, Kingston, Ontario, Health Guide Series.

Gerard S. Upton, Patientologist, "Graves' Eye Disease: A Patient's Point of View" (*Thyrobulletin*, Winter 1992).

Robert Volpé, M.D., interviewed, 1991.

Dr. Jack Wall, "Thyroid-Associated Ophthalmopathy from the Investigator's Point of View" (*Thyrobulletin*, Spring 1992).

Lawrence C. Wood, M.D., F.A.C.P., David S. Cooper, M.D., F.A.C.P., and E. Chester Ridgway, M.D., F.A.C.P., *Your Thyroid: A Home Reference* (1990, Ballantine Books, New York).

Chapter 4

H. Jack Baskin, M.D., *How Your Thyroid Works, 3rd ed.* (1991, Adams Press, Chicago).

R. I. S. Bayliss and W. M. G. Tunbridge, *Thyroid Disease: The Facts* (1991, Oxford University Press, New York).

Joel I. Hamburger, M.D., F.A.C.P., *The Thyroid Gland: A Book For Thyroid Patients, 7th ed.* (1991, Joel Hamburger, M.D., Southfield, Michigan).

"Thyroiditis," National Headquarters, Thyroid Foundation of Canada, Kingston, Ontario, Health Guide Series.

Lawrence C. Wood, M.D., F.A.C.P., David S. Cooper, M.D., F.A.C.P., and E. Chester Ridgway, M.D., F.A.C.P., *Your Thyroid: A Home Reference* (1990, Ballantine Books, New York).

Chapter 5

H. Jack Baskin, M.D., *How Your Thyroid Works, 3rd ed.* (1991, Adams Press, Chicago).

R. I. S. Bayliss and W. M. G. Tunbridge, *Thyroid Disease: The Facts* (1991, Oxford University Press, New York).

Dorland's Illustrated Medical Dictionary, 26th ed. (1981, W. B. Saunders Company, Philadelphia).

Joel I. Hamburger, M.D., F.A.C.P., *The Thyroid Gland: A Book For Thyroid Patients, 7th ed.* (1991, Joel Hamburger, M.D., Southfield, Michigan).

Dr. Timothy O'Leary, "Needle Biopsy: A New Technique for Thyroid Nodules" (*Thyrobulletin*, Summer 1989).

Irving B. Rosen, M.D., F.R.C.S. (C), F.A.C.S., Associate Professor, Department of Surgery, University of Toronto, Mount Sinai Hospital, "The Thyroid Operation: A Patient's Perspective" (Lecture presented to Thyroid Foundation of Canada, October 1991).

———, interviewed, October 1991.

"Thyroid Nodules," National Headquarters, Thyroid Foundation of Canada, Kingston, Ontario, Health Guide Series.

Lawrence C. Wood, M.D., F.A.C.P., David S. Cooper, M.D., F.A.C.P., and E. Chester Ridgway, M.D., F.A.C.P., *Your Thyroid: A Home Reference* (1990, Ballantine Books, New York).

Chapter 6

H. Jack Baskin, M.D., *How Your Thyroid Works, 3rd ed.* (1991, Adams Press, Chicago).

R. I. S. Bayliss and W. M. G. Tunbridge, *Thyroid Disease: The Facts* (1991, Oxford University Press, New York).

Dorland's Illustrated Medical Dictionary, 26th ed. (1981, W. B. Saunders Company, Philadelphia).

"Facts on Thyroid Cancer" (Canadian Cancer Society, December 1986.)

"Guidelines for Patients Receiving Radioiodine Treatment" (Society of Nuclear Medicine, New York).

Joel I. Hamburger, M.D., F.A.C.P., *The Thyroid Gland: A Book For Thyroid Patients, 7th ed.* (1991, Joel Hamburger, M.D., Southfield, Michigan).

"If You Received X-Ray Treatment to Your Head or Neck Area as a Child Or Young Adult..." (Canadian Cancer Society, 1981).

Irving B. Rosen, M.D., F.R.C.S. (C), F.A.C.S., Associate Professor, Department of Surgery, University of Toronto, Mount Sinai Hosital, "The Thyroid Operation: A Patient's Perspective," (Lecture presented to Thyroid Foundation of Canada, October 1991).

———, interviewed, October 1991.

Dr. Lorne Rotstein, Assistant Professor of Surgery, University of Toronto; Chief, General Surgical Oncology, Toronto Hospital, "Cancer Surgery," from *Surgery, A Complete Guide for Patients and Their Families*, Allan Gross, M.D., Penny Gross, Ph.D., and Bernard Langer, M.D., eds., University of Toronto Department of Surgery (1989, HarperCollins, Toronto).

"Thyroid Nodules," National Headquarters, Thyroid Foundation of Canada, Kingston, Ontario, Health Guide Series.

Lawrence C. Wood, M.D., F.A.C.P., David S. Cooper, M.D., F.A.C.P., and E. Chester Ridgway, M.D., F.A.C.P., *Your Thyroid: A Home Reference* (1990, Ballantine Books, New York).

Chapter 7

H. Jack Baskin, M.D., *How Your Thyroid Works, 3rd ed.* (1991, Adams Press, Chicago).

R. I. S. Bayliss and W. M. G. Tunbridge, *Thyroid Disease: The Facts* (1991, Oxford University Press, New York).

Gregory P. Becks, M.D., F.R.C.P., and Gerard N. Burrow, M.D., F.R.C.P. (C), "Thyroid Disorders and Pregnancy" (*The Bridge*, Vol. 4, No. 3).

Joel I. Hamburger, M.D., F.A.C.P., *The Thyroid Gland: A Book for Thyroid Patients, 7th ed.* (1991, Joel Hamburger, M.D., Southfield, Michigan).

Dr. R. W. Hudson, "The Effects of Thyroid Hormone on Reproductive Function" (*Thyrobulletin*, Autumn 1990).

Mark Patry, M.D., "The Thyroid and Menopause" (*Thyrobulletin*, Summer 1991).

Irving B. Rosen, M.D., F.R.C.S. (C), F.A.C.S., Associate Professor, Department of Surgery, University of Toronto, Mount Sinai Hospital, "The Thyroid Operation: A Patient's Perspective" (Lecture presented to Thyroid Foundation of Canada, October 1991).

———, interviewed, October 1991.

"Thyroid Disease, Pregnancy and Fertility," National Headquarters, Thyroid Foundation of Canada, Kingston, Ontario, Health Guide Series.

Lawrence C. Wood, M.D., F.A.C.P., David S. Cooper, M.D., F.A.C.P., and E. Chester Ridgway, M.D., F.A.C.P., *Your Thyroid: A Home Reference* (1990, Ballantine Books, New York).

Chapter 8

Dr. R. W. Hudson, "The Effects of Thyroid Hormone on Reproductive Function" (*Thyrobulletin*, Autumn 1990).

John Pimenoff, Patient, interviewed, 1992.

Irving B. Rosen, M.D., F.R.C.S. (C), F.A.C.S., Associate Professor, Department of Surgery, University of Toronto, Mount Sinai Hospital, "The Thyroid Operation: A Patient's Perspective" (Lecture presented to Thyroid Foundation of Canada, October 1991).

———, interviewed, October 1991.

Chapter 9

H. Jack Baskin, M.D., *How Your Thyroid Works, 3rd ed.* (1991, Adams Press, Chicago).

R. I. S. Bayliss and W. M. G. Tunbridge, *Thyroid Disease: The Facts* (1991, Oxford University Press, New York).

Gregory P. Becks, M.D., F.R.C.P., and Gerard N. Burrow, M.D., F.R.C.P. (C), "Thyroid Disorders and Pregnancy" (*The Bridge*, Vol. 4, No. 3).

Marilyn Dunlop, "What's New In Medicine" (*The Toronto Star*, November 7, 1992).

Joel I. Hamburger, M.D., F.A.C.P., *The Thyroid Gland: A Book For Thyroid Patients, 7th ed.* (1991, Joel Hamburger, M.D., Southfield, Michigan).

Dr. R. W. Hudson, "The Effects of Thyroid Hormone on Reproductive Function" (*Thyrobulletin*, Autumn 1990).

Matthew Lazar, M.D., F.R.C.P. (C), F.A.A.P., Pediatrician, interviewed, 1993.

"Newborn Screening: Ensuring a Healthy Start" (Ontario Ministry of Health, 1981).

"Thyroid Disease, Pregnancy and Fertility," "Thyroid Disease in Childhood," Thyroid Foundation of Canada, Kingston, Ontario, Health Guide Series.

Lawrence C. Wood, M.D., F.A.C.P., David S. Cooper, M.D., F.A.C.P., and E. Chester Ridgway, M.D., F.A.C.P., *Your Thyroid: A Home Reference* (1990, Ballantine Books, New York).

Chapter 10

Heather R. Dawson, M.D., C.C.F.P., Family Practitioner; Assistant Professor, University of Toronto, interviewed, 1991.

Janet Maurer, M.D., *How to Talk to Your Doctor: The Questions to Ask* (1986, Simon & Schuster, Inc., New York).

Chapter 11

H. Jack Baskin, M.D., *How Your Thyroid Works, 3rd ed.* (1991, Adams Press, Chicago).

R. I. S. Bayliss and W. M. G. Tunbridge, *Thyroid Disease: The Facts* (1991, Oxford University Press, New York).

David Becker, M.D. "Chernobyl: The Accident and Its Implications" (*Thyrobulletin*, Autumn 1990).

Dr. Ted Cross, "The Use of Radioactive Iodine" (Lecture presented to Thyroid Foundation of Canada, March 1992).

"Guidelines for Patients Receiving Radioiodine Treatment" (Society of Nuclear Medicine, New York, 1983).

Joel I. Hamburger, M.D., F.A.C.P., *The Thyroid Gland: A Book for Thyroid Patients, 7th ed.* (1991, Joel Hamburger, M.D., Southfield, Michigan).

Daniel Rappaport, M.D., F.R.C.P. (C), Radiologist, interviewed, 1991.

"Thyroid Nodules," National Headquarters, Thyroid Foundation of Canada, Kingston, Ontario, Health Guide Series.

Lawrence C. Wood, M.D., F.A.C.P., David S. Cooper, M.D., F.A.C.P., and E. Chester Ridgway, M.D., F.A.C.P., *Your Thyroid: A Home Reference* (1990, Ballantine Books, New York).

Chapter 12

"Dyes and Drugs: Interactions and Cautions" (*Thyrobulletin*, Autumn 1989).

"Dyes and Drugs Update: No Danger" (*Thyrobulletin*, Spring 1990).

"For the Hypothyroid Patient" (Distributor: Glaxo, 1992).

"Medications for Hypothyroidism" (Thyroid Foundation of Canada, December 1990).

Bob Pritchard, Pharmacist, Coordinator, Public and Professional Information for Shoppers, Drugmart Pharmacies, Ltd.; interviewed, 1991.

Chapter 13

M. C. Goldenberg, M.D., F.R.C.P. (C), "Thyroid Disease Late in Life," (Lecture presented to Thyroid Foundation of Canada, April 8, 1987.)

Ian R. Hart, F.R.C.P. (C), "Thyroid Research 1985" (Distributed by Thyroid Foundation of Canada).

Susan MacNeil, R.P.Dt., "Nutrition and the Thyroid" (Lecture presented to Thyroid Foundation of Canada, April 14, 1987).

"Thyroid Research in Canada" (Special Issue, *Thyrobulletin*, Summer 1992).

"Thyroid Disease in Late Life," National Headquarters, Thyroid Foundation of Canada, Kingston, Ontario, Health Guide Series.

Note: Thyroid Foundation of Canada Health Guides were written by Drs. Ian R. Hart, Robert Volpé, Paul G. Walfish, and Jack R. Wall.

Additional Resources for the Second Edition

"Are all Nodules Cancerous?" Patient information supplied by The Thyroid Society for Education and Research, 1992.

"Autoimmune Thyroid Diseases" (*Thyroid Signpost*, Volume 1, Number 5, August 1993).

Beardall, Ross A., Thyroid Disease in Pets. (*Thyrobulletin*, Volume 16, Number 2, Summer 1995).

Becker, David, M.D., "Radiation and the Thyroid" (*Thyrobulletin*, Volume 16, Number 3, Autumn 1995).

Benvenga, Salvatore, Luigi Bartolone, Stefano Squadrito, Francesco lo Giudice, and Francesco Trimarchi, "Delayed Intestinal Absorption of Levothyroixine" (*Thyroid*, Volume 5, Number 4, August 1995).

"Blood Test Detect Thyroid Cancer Gene" (*Thyrobulletin*, Volume 16, Number 1, Spring 1995).

Bogdanova, Tatyana, I., Ph.D., and Nikolaj D. Tranko, M.D., Ph.D, Institute of Endocrinology and Metabolism, Academy of Medical Sciences of Ukraine, Kiev, Ukraine. "The Dynamics of Thyroid Cancer in Children in Ukraine After the Chernobyl Accident." Unpublished as of this writing.

Bogner, U., et al., "Association between thyroid cytotoxic antibodies and atrophic thyroiditis" (*Clinical Thyroidology*, Volume VIII, Issue 1, January–April 1995).

"Cholesterol and Thyroid Disease" (*Thyroid Signpost*, Volume 1, Number 2, May 1993).

Clark, Orlo H., M.D., and Johann Elmhed, "Thyroid Surgery—Past, Present, and Future" (*Thyroid Today*, Volume XVIII, Number 1, March 1995).

Cooper, David S., M.D., "Thyroid Nodules and Thyroid Cancer: Evaluation and Treatment" (*Thyrobulletin*, Volume 16, Number 3, Autumn 1995).

Daniels, Gilbert H., M.D., "Graves' Eye Disease" (*Thyrobulletin*, Volume 15, Number 4, January 1995).

Davies, Terry F., M.D., F.R.C.P., "New Thinking on the Immunology of Graves' Disease" (*Thyroid Today*, Volume XV, Number 4, 1992).

Delange, F., Executive Director, International Council for Control of Iodine Deficiency Disorders. "Iodine Deficiency Disorders and Their Prevention: A Worldwide Problem." Abstract from the 6th International Thyroid Symposium, Thyroid and Trace Elements, 1996.

"Depression and Thyroid Disease" (*Thyroid Signpost*, Volume 1, Number 3, June 1993).

Dirusso, G., et al., "Complications of I-131 Radioablation for Well-Differentiated Thyroid Cancer" (*Clinical Thyroidology*, Volume VIII, Issue 1, January–April 1995).

Dottorini, M.E., et al. "Effect of Radioiodine for Thyroid Cancer on Carcinogenesis and Female Fertility" (*Clinical Thyroidology*, Volume VIII, Issue 1, January-April 1995).

Eskin, B. A., Medical College of Pennsylvania and Hahnemann University, Philadelphia, Penn. "Effects of Iodine Therapy on Breast Cancer and the Thyroid." Abstract from the 6th International Thyroid Symposium, Thyroid and Trace Elements, 1996.

Gaitan, Eduardo, M.D., F.A.C., "Goiter" (*The Bridge*, Volume 10, Number 3, Fall 1995).

Garton, M., et al., "Effect of L-Thyroxine Replacement on Bone Mineral Density and Metabolism in Premenopausal Women" (*Clinical Thyroidology*, Volume VIII, Issue 1, January–April 1995).

Gaz, Randall D., M.D., "Instructions for Patients Undergoing Thyroid Needle Biopsy" (*Thyrobulletin*, Volume 14, Number 4, Autumn 1993).

Ginsberg, Jody, M.D., F.R.C.P., "Wilson's Syndrome and T3" (*Thyrobulletin*, Volume 15, Number 4, January 1995).

Glinoer, D., M.D., Ph.D., "The Thyroid Gland and Pregnancy: Iodine Restriction and Goitrogenesis Revealed" *(Thyroid International* 5, 1994).

"Graves' Eye Disease" (*Thyroid Signpost*, Volume 1, Number 6, September 1993).

"Hair Loss and Thyroid Disease" (*Thyroid Signpost*, Volume 1, Number 1, April 1993).

Hart, Ian R., M.B., Ch.B. M.Sc., F.R.C.P.C., F.A.C.P., F.R.C.P., (Glas), "Does Your Patient Have a Thyroid Problem?" (*Medicine North America*, February 1996).

Havas, S., and J. M. Hershman, West Los Angeles VA Medical Center, UCLA, Los Angeles, Calif., "Action of Lithium on the Thyroid." Abstract from the 6th International Thyroid Symposium, Thyroid and Trace Elements, 1996.

Hetzel, Basil S., M.D., Chairman, International Council for Control of Iodine Deficiency Disorders, North Adelaide, Australia, "Iodine Deficiency and Excess: A World Problem" (*Thyrobulletin*, Volume 16, Number 3, Autumn 1995).

Horn-Ross, P. L., A. S. Whittemore, D. W. West, and I. R. McDougall., Northern California Cancer Center, Union City, Calif., "Rationale for a Study of Iodine, Selenium and Thyroid Cancer." Abstract from the 6th International Thyroid Symposium, Thyroid and Trace Elements, 1996.

Ito, Masahiro, et al., "Childhood Thyroid Diseases Around Chernobyl Evaluated by Ultrasound Examination and Fine Needle Aspiration Cytology" (*Thyroid*, Volume 5, Number 5, 1995).

Loebig, Poertl H., et al., Division of Endocrinology, Department of Medicine, University of Essen, Essen and Department of Medicine, University of Bochum, Bochum, Germany. "Regulation of Maternal Thyroid During Pregnancy by Human Chorionic Gonadotropin (hCG)." Abstract from the 6th International Thyroid Symposium, Thyroid and Trace Elements, 1996.

Martino, E., et al., "Increased Susceptibility to Hypothyroidism in Patients with Autoimmune Thyroid Disease Treated with Amiodarone" (*Clinical Thyroidology*, Volume VIII, Issue 1, January–April 1995).

Matoo, T. K., "Primary Hypothyroidism Ecodary to Nephrotic Syndrome in Infancy" (*Clinical Thyroidology*, Volume VIII, Issue 1, January–April 1995).

Mitchell, Marvin L., M.D., "Congenital Hypothyroidism" (*The Bridge*, Volume 10, Number 4, Winter 1995).

Nygaard, B., et al., "Acute Effects of Radioiodine Therapy on Thyroid Gland Size and Function in Patients with Multinodular Goiter" (*Clinical Thyroidology*, Volume VIII, Issue 1, January-April 1995).

O'Riordain, D. S., et al., "Impact of Biochemical Screening of Medullary Thyroid Cancer: Extent of Disease and Outcome in Patients with Multiple Endocrine Neoplasia" (*Clinical Thyroidology*, Volume VIII, Issue 1, January–April 1995).

Perros, P., et al, "Natural History of Thyroid Associated Ophthalmopathy" (*Clinical Thyroidology*, Volume VIII, Issue 1, January–April 1995).

Reiners, Chr., Clinic and Policlinic for Nuclear Medicine, University of Wurzburg, Germany. "Radioactive Iodine and the Risk of Thyroid Cancer." Abstract from the 6th International Thyroid Symposium, Thyroid and Trace Elements, 1996.

Rosen, Irving B., M.D., F.R.C.S.C., F.A.C.S., and Paul Walfish, CM, M.D., F.R.C.P.C., F.A.C.P., F.R.S.M., "You and Thyroid Cancer" (*Thyrobulletin*, Volume 16, Number 4, January 1996).

Rosenthal, M. Sara, *The Breast Sourcebook* (1996, Lowell House, Los Angeles).

———, *The Fertility Sourcebook* (1996, Lowell House, Los Angeles).

———, *The Gynecological Sourcebook* (1995, Lowell House, Los Angeles).

Ross, Douglas S., M.D., "Fine Needle Aspiration Biopsy of Thyroid Nodules" (*Thyrobulletin*, Volume 14, Number 4, Autumn 1993).

Singer, Peter A., M.D., "Hashimoto's Thyroiditis" (*Thyrobulletin*, Volume 16, Number 1, Spring 1995).

Singh, A., et al., "Thyroid Antibodies as a Predictor of Early Reproductive Failure" (*Clinical Thyroidology*, Volume VIII, Issue 1, January–April 1995).

Solomon, Diane, M.D., "Fine Needle Aspiration of the Thyroid: an Update" (*Thyroid Today*, Volume XVI, Number 3, September 1993).

"Solving the Puzzle of Thyroid Therapy." Physician literature, supplied by Knoll Pharma Inc., 1995.

Surks, Martin I., M.D., *The Thyroid Book* (1994, Consumer Reports Books, Yonkers, New York).

"TED (Thyroid Eye Disease)." Patient information leaflet, supplied by TED, 1995.

"The Facts About Thyroid Nodules." Patient literature, supplied by Daniels Pharmaceuticals, Inc., 1995.

"The Many Aspects of Subclinical Hypothyroidism." Physician literature, supplied by Knoll Pharma Inc., 1995.

"The Many Faces of Undiagnosed Hypothyroidism." Physician literature, supplied by Knoll Pharma Inc., 1995.

"Thyroid Disease and Osteoporosis." Patient information leaflet, supplied by the British Thyroid Foundation and the National Osteoporosis Society, 1992.

"To Confirm the Clinical Diagnosis." Patient information, supplied by the British Thyroid Foundation, 1992.

"Treatment Options for Hyperthyroidism and Graves' Disease" (*Thyroid Signpost*, Volume 1, Number 4, July 1993).

Toft, Anthony D., M.D., "Other Forms of Hyperthyroidism" (*Thyrobulletin*, Volume 16, Number 3, Autumn 1995).

Tuttle, R. Michael, Troy Patience, and Steven Budd, "Treatment with Propylthiouracil Before Radioactive Iodine Therapy is Associated with a Higher Treatment Failure Rate than Therapy with Radioactive Iodine Alone in Graves' Disease" (*Thyroid*, Volume 5, Number 4, August 1995).

VanMiddlesworth, L. Department of Physiology, University of Tennessee, Memphis, Tenn., "Usual and Unusual Isotopes in the Thyroid." Abstract from the 6th International Thyroid Symposium, Thyroid and Trace Elements, 1996.

Varl, B., J. Drinovec, and M. Bagar-Posve, Research Unit Radenska Redenci, zdravilisko naselje 14, 69252, Radeci, Slovenia. "Iodine Supply with Mineral Water." Abstract from the 6th International Thyroid Symposium, Thyroid and Trace Elements, 1996.

Walfish, Paul, M.D., "Thyroid Disease During and After Pregnancy" (*Thyrobulletin*, Volume 16, Number 3, Autumn 1995).

Wesche, M. F., et al., "Long-term effect of radioiodine therapy on goiter size in patients with nontoxic multinodular goiter" (*Clinical Thyroidology*, Volume VIII, Issue 1, January–April 1995).

"What About Tests and Treatment?" Patient information, supplied by The Thyroid Society for Education and Research, 1992.

"What is Hyperthyroidism?" Patient information, supplied by The Thyroid Society for Education and Research, 1992.

"What is Hypothyroidism?" Patient information, supplied by The Thyroid Society for Education and Research, 1992.

"What is Thyroid Disease?" Patient information, supplied by The Thyroid Society for Education and Research, 1992.

"What is Thyroiditis?" Patient information, supplied by The Thyroid Society for Education and Research, 1992.

Wood, Lawrence C., M.D., David S. Cooper, M.D., and E. Chester Ridgway, M.D., *Your Thyroid: A Home Reference, 3rd ed.* (1995, Ballantine Books, New York).

Index

NSAIDS (nonsteroidal anti-inflammatory drugs), 19
Nutrition, 224-231
  and calories, 225
  dietary fat reduction, 227-228
  for euthyroidism, 227
  food for hyperthyroidism, 225-226
  food for hypothyroidism, 226-227
  good fats/bad fats, 228-231
  trimming the fat, 230-231

Oophorectomy defined, 119
Oral contraception, 108-109
Orbital decompression, 49
Osteoporosis, 121-122
  menopause and thyroid issues, 122
  preventing, 122
Outpatients, 221-222

Pain, non-cyclical breast, 118
Papillary cancer, 86-87
Papillary-follicular mix, 87
Parathyroid glands, 8-9
Patients, bill of rights of, 161-163
Patients, problems reporting symptoms to doctor, 157
Periods, menstrual, 107-108
Pernicious anemia, 55-56
Pharmacists
  choosing, 218-220
  problems of, 215-218
  using, 214-220
Physicians; See Doctors
Pituitary glands, 6
Pituitary-thyroid regulating system, 40
Plummer's syndrome, 26-27
Postpartum hypothyroidism, 37
Postpartum thyroid disease, 66
Postpartum thyroiditis, 60, 64-67, 106, 111, 117
  diagnosing, 65-66
  treating, 66
Posttreatment precautions, 187-188
Potassium iodide, 194-197
Pregnancy, 111-117
  and the baby's thyroid, 113

finding a thyroid nodule in, 116
and normal thyroid function, 112-113
planning one's, 111-112
and postpartum thyroid disease, 116-117
thyroid disease during, 113-116
Pregnancy Sourcebook, The, 67, 111, 189
Premarin, 120
Progesterone-only contraception, 109
Prolactin, 107
Pronounced anemia, 226
Prophylactic thyroidectomy, 88
PTU (propylthiouracil), 66, 115-116, 118, 212
Pulse, taking one's, 39

Quervain's thyroiditis, 61-63

RA (rheumatoid arthritis), 56-57
Radiation, external, 98-101
Radioactive iodine 27, 29-30, 50, 112, 181-197; See also Nonradioactive iodine
  affects on healthy children, 85
  affects on healthy thyroids, 191-197
  and Chernobyl, 192-194
  defined, 181-182
  exposure to fallout, 195-196
  imaging tests, 184-185
  layperson's guide to, 181-197
  myths, 189-191
  and potassium iodide, 194-197
  thyroid testing, 182-185
  treatment, 95, 115, 148-149, 185-191
  update tests, 183-184
Reagan, Ronald, 128
Reproduction, male, 131-132
Research
  1995: year of the thyroid, 233-234
  and the developed world, 232-233
  funding, 233
  on the horizon, 231-236
  and technology, 235-236
  and the underdeveloped world, 232
Riedel's thyroiditis, 67-68